Suicide Prevention

T0262601

Suicide Prevention

Christine Yu Moutier

Chief Medical Officer, The American Foundation for Suicide Prevention

Anthony R. Pisani

Associate Professor of Psychiatry and Pediatrics
University of Rochester Medical Center, New York

Stephen M. Stahl

Professor of Psychiatry and Neuroscience, University of California at
Riverside and San Diego

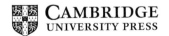

CAMBRIDGE
UNIVERSITY PRESS

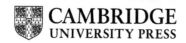

Shaftesbury Road, Cambridge CB2 8EA, United Kingdom

One Liberty Plaza, 20th Floor, New York, NY 10006, USA

477 Williamstown Road, Port Melbourne, VIC 3207, Australia

314–321, 3rd Floor, Plot 3, Splendor Forum, Jasola District Centre, New Delhi – 110025, India

103 Penang Road, #05–06/07, Visioncrest Commercial, Singapore 238467

Cambridge University Press is part of Cambridge University Press & Assessment, a department of the University of Cambridge.

We share the University's mission to contribute to society through the pursuit of education, learning and research at the highest international levels of excellence.

www.cambridge.org
Information on this title: www.cambridge.org/9781108463621
DOI: 10.1017/9781108564618

First published 2021 (version 4, February 2023)

Printed in the United Kingdom by TJ Books Limited, Padstow Cornwall

A catalogue record for this publication is available from the British Library

ISBN 978-1-108-46362-1 Paperback

Contents

Acknowledgements

Dr. Moutier:

I'd like to acknowledge my colleagues who have laid much of the scientific foundation for the clinical guidance provided in this handbook. For providing me with personal encouragement and inspiration, and for your deep and longstanding dedication to suicide prevention, I am grateful for each of you – Drs. Sidney Zisook, Yeates Conwell, Maria Oquendo, John Mann, Jill Harkavy-Friedman, Doreen Marshall, David Brent, Joan Asarnow, Barbara Stanley, Greg Brown, Dave Jobes, Jerry Rosenbaum, Gretchen Haas, Peter Marzuk, Gary Kennedy, Kathy Shear, Lisa Horowitz, Maddy Gould, David Gunnell, Gil Zalsman, Caitlin Ryan, Rory O'Connor, David Covington, Emmy Betz, Guy Diamond. To the many patients, trainees, colleagues, friends, and family who have opened yourselves up and disclosed your suicidal struggles and experiences of loss – I have learned from you even as I have tried my best to use my own clinical and lived experience to support you. To my colleague, Alex McRae, thank you for providing immeasurable support in preparation of this manuscript. And to my co-authors: Dr. Tony Pisani, I needed your deep expertise in primary care and as an NIH-funded developer and evaluator of suicide prevention efforts across many clinical settings. I appreciate that you were game to collaborate. Lastly, Dr. Stephen Stahl, your generous partnership and desire to help clinicians prevent suicide has been genuinely evident – thank you.

Dr. Pisani:

I would like to acknowledge my close collaborator, Kristina Mossgraber, lived experience faculty at SafeSide Prevention and one of the coolest people I know. Things Kristina has said or taught me permeate every page I wrote. My longtime editor and friend, Paul Scade, helped me capture both the skills and the heart behind the clinical framework I use and teach. I'm grateful for this author team. Christine Moutier is on a mission. Gifted communicator, brilliant strategist, and wise confidante, Christine inspires me every time we're together. Steve Stahl has a knack for understanding and providing exactly what health professionals need to do our job better. It was a privilege to learn how he thinks, and to join this practical book series which has touched so many lives.

Dr. Stahl:

With gratitude to my coauthors Christine Moutier and Anthony Pisani for imparting their wisdom in a practical way to reach readers. With praise for our editor Catherine Barnes at Cambridge University Press for facilitating publication of this important handbook.

SECTION 1
Suicide Prevention Overview

1

Translating Science into Action

Ⓐ Introduction: Science, Culture, and Readiness to Act

The current scientifically informed view of suicide is that, while complex, suicide is a health-related outcome. Driven by a convergence of health factors along with other psychosocial and environmental factors, suicide risk is multifactorial. Like most health outcomes, a set of genetic, environmental, and psychological/behavioral factors are relevant. It is critically important that health professionals develop a current understanding of suicide as older views have permeated and clouded societal understanding leading to assumptions and judgment that have silenced generations of people suffering suicidal struggles or loss of a loved one to suicide.

Evolving attitudes toward suicide are not limited to the scientific or medical field. Science is impacting popular culture as well. Recent polls in the USA show that public perceptions of mental health and suicide are changing quite rapidly toward greater awareness, open-mindedness, and diminishing stigma.[1] For example, 90% of respondents believe that mental health is as valid and important as physical health, and say they would help if someone they know were to become suicidal. However many add they are not necessarily equipped with skills and language to know how to help.

Key Point
Suicide, while complex, is a health-related outcome.

Figures 1.1, 1.2, 1.3 Examples of positively evolving attitudes toward mental health and suicide prevention among the American public

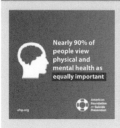
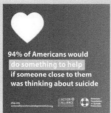
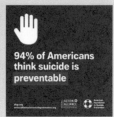

New attitudes toward mental health in general and suicide in particular are reflected in the growing suicide prevention movement that has emerged in recent years in the USA, UK, Australia, and other nations. The truth is that for millennia, people who had lost loved ones and people who experienced a loved one's suicidal crisis or their own largely kept their experiences to themselves, but now are speaking out and are part of leading the movement to advance change. Advocates on all sides of the issue have come together to raise public awareness, to advocate for changes in national policy for increases in research funding, improved healthcare access, for enforcement of mental health parity, and to call for an end to discriminatory practices in school and workplace settings. This public movement has led to hundreds of thousands of people participating in events in the USA such as the Out of the Darkness Walks for suicide prevention in all 50 states, advocacy activities at state and federal levels, and educational programs on how to prevent and respond to suicide in workplaces, schools, and faith-based settings.

The bottom line is that in today's environment, healthcare providers need not be hesitant to address mental health concerns with their patients. The truth is that many patients may be open to dialog and in need of support but 1) may not be sure if their health provider will respond in a compassionate and knowledgeable way related to suicidal thoughts or mental health concerns, and 2) they may not know how to bring up their symptoms or concerns and may not have sophisticated language for symptoms. But even with these concerns present or with current robust mental health, many patients appreciate having their mental health screened and addressed in a manner similar to physical health.

While culture and attitudes toward mental health are opening up, it is a time of transition in culture and belief systems with natural unevenness to the pace and regionality of changing views. Thus, in general, the public's level of mental health literacy in terms of when and how to take action remains relatively low.[2] Health professionals can help deepen their patients' understanding of mental health in the same way they do for physical health. As is the case for many physical health targets such as cardiovascular health, for patients who carry any degree of elevated risk, patient education, clinical treatment, family support, and personalized lifestyle habits can improve prognosis and change outcomes.

Key Point
Patients appreciate having their mental health addressed in a similar manner as their physical health. Routine health maintenance in primary care should include mental health and suicide risk reduction. For all health professionals, basic principles included in this handbook will facilitate caring, competent handling of patients who are at risk for suicide.

B PRINCIPLES

- From a public health perspective, suicide is considered a generally preventable cause of death. This does not mean all suicides can be prevented, or that suicide is a predictable event.

- Health systems and providers across disciplines have a vital role to play in suicide prevention.

- The combination of scientific discovery and voices of people with lived experience and loss is advancing culture change and a new societal readiness when it comes to suicide prevention.

- Cultural norms in many regions of the world are changing in relation to mental health and suicide, with people beginning to open up and speak out about mental health, reducing the stigma around mental health, help seeking, and suicide prevention.

- While the absolute number of suicides around the globe has been on the rise since 2000, the overall rate has been decreasing as the world's population grows.

- Suicide risk is complex and multi-faceted for individuals and for populations.

- A multi-pronged approach is needed to prevent suicide in a population. Efforts must include basic public health strategies such as universal education, community based initiatives, effective and available clinical care, and better surveillance of suicide attempts and deaths.

- Other critical components of an effective suicide prevention effort are investments in research and the development of new suicide prevention focused treatments for clinical use.

- Federal and local investments in suicide prevention research, community programs, and clinical treatments can reduce suicide mortality.

Key Concept "Prevention" versus "Prediction"
- Research shows that suicide can be prevented.
- From a public health perspective, suicide is considered a generally preventable cause of death.
- This does not mean all suicides can be prevented, nor that suicide is a predictable event.
- In the same way that death due to myocardial infarction is not a predictable event on the individual patient level or with a pinpoint on the timing or severity of an event, but cardiologists and primary care understand that aggressively addressing risk factors of cardiovascular disease can save lives. The same principles are true for suicide.
- Lack of predictability does not mean a health outcome is not preventable by using upstream, population health approaches, in addition to individualized clinical interventions and family/peer strategies.

 Scope of the Problem and Trends

● **Global Perspective**

We are living in a time of pressing urgency: suicide is a global problem, a leading cause of death with a staggering loss of 800,000 lives each year. Suicide cuts across high- and low-income countries, with lower- and middle-income countries bearing the largest burden (80% of all suicides), but with suicide continuing to be a serious problem in high-income countries as well. In recent years, the World Health Organization (WHO) and the United Nations (UN) have adopted action plans focused on mental health and suicide prevention, and have set goals to reduce the rate of suicide by 10% by 2020 in the case of WHO and by 33% by 2030 in the case of the UN Sustainable Development Goals.[3] Presently, 40 countries have enacted national strategies to prevent suicide,[4] several of which are proving effective, with reductions in suicide rates in many countries such as China, Denmark, England, Switzerland, the Philippines, and South Korea.[5] And although the absolute number of suicides globally continues to increase, a recent study accounting for population growth found the global rate of suicide has dropped by 32.7% over the past three decades.[5]

Key Point
Suicide is a global health problem and a national priority for many countries.

Figure 1.4 WHO global map of suicide rates by region of the world

National suicide rates vary widely throughout the world. Illustrated by color coding with darker colors showing the countries with higher suicide rates, this map shows the variability across nations. It is important to note that some countries' suicide data is more accurate than others related to the complexity of vital statistics and death investigation systems as well as the variability of the approach and progress between countries. See Figure 1.7 for more information about countries' quality of vital statistics and suicide data.

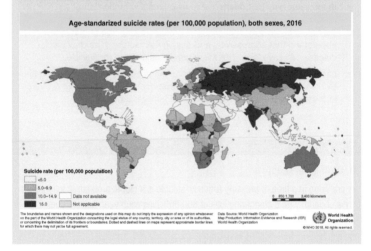

Age-standarized suicide rates (per 100,000 population), both sexes, 2016

Suicide rate (per 100,000 population)

- <5.0
- 5.0–9.9
- 10.0–14.9   Data not available
- 15.0   Not applicable

0   850 1,700   3,400 kilometers

The boundaries and names shown and the designations used on this map do not imply the expression of any opinion whatsoever on the part of the World Health Organization concerning the legal status of any country, territory, city or area or of its authorities, or concerning the delimitation of its frontiers or boundaries. Dotted and dashed lines on maps represent approximate border lines for which there may not yet be full agreement.

Data Source: World Health Organization
Map Production: Information Evidence and Research (IER)
World Health Organization

World Health Organization

Figure 1.5 Suicide rates in several nations (1990–2017)

Note the world suicide rate shown by the green line. While the absolute number of suicides around the globe has been on the rise, the rate has been decreasing as the world's population grows. Several countries' suicide rates have remained stable (e.g., Greece), several are decreasing (e.g., UK, Germany), and the USA is one of few whose national suicide rate is steadily increasing since 1999.

Suicide death rates

Age-standardized death rates from suicide, measured as the number of deaths per 100,000 individuals.
Age-standardization assumes a constant population age and structure to allow for comparisons between countries
and with time without the effects of a changing age distribution within a population (e.g., aging).

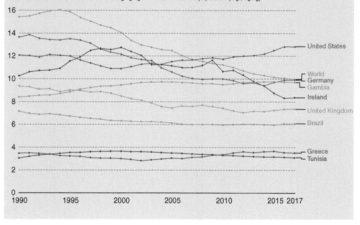

Note the scale of the y-axis which is multiple-fold that of the previous graph. Lithuania, Guyana, and South Korea have some of the highest known suicide rates around the globe. South Korea has seen a significant decrease in their national rate over the past decade of 15% after the leading pesticide was banned by law in 2011.

Suicide death rates

Suicide death rates are measured as the number of deaths per 100,000 individuals in a given population.

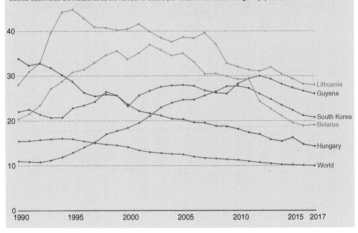

Figure 1.7 WHO global map showing quality of vital registration data

The quality and reliability of suicide data is highly variable across nations. According to WHO, of its 172 Member States, which publish suicide estimates, only 80 have reasonably good quality vital registration data systems to collect suicide data.

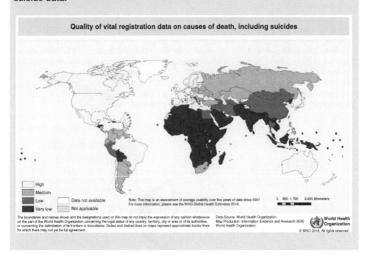

One caveat regarding international suicide data is that data is deficient for two reasons: not all countries have reliable systems in place to collect quality vital registration data including suicide data; additionally stigma and complexities of medical and legal systems involved in data collection make the reported numbers variable in their accuracy as well.[6] Without solid data tracked as close to real time as possible, it is challenging to measure the success of suicide prevention and intervention strategies. This highlights the importance of surveillance as part of any effective suicide prevention plan, and applies to nations, but certainly applies to health systems as well. See Chapter 10 for steps health systems can take to prevent suicide, including developing ways to track attempts and suicide deaths.

D **Public Health Model of Suicide Includes the Full Continuum of Experience from Suicidal Ideation to Attempts to Death and Loss**

 Figure 1.8 The scope of the public health crisis of suicide includes ideation, attempts, and suicide loss.

The approach to suicide prevention must include consideration of the millions of individuals who experience upstream distress including suicidal thoughts and behaviors, as well as those bereaved by suicide. In the USA estimates by the Substance Abuse and Mental Health Services Administration (SAMHSA) are that 1.4 million American adults attempt suicide each year and approximately 12 million seriously consider suicide. A total of 51% of adults know someone who died by suicide during their lifetime.[7] A strong public health approach considers the needs of all of these experiences. National Institute of Mental Health (NIMH), www.nimh.nih.gov/health/statistics/suicide.shtml#part_155013

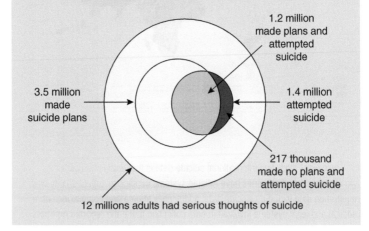

1.2 million made plans and attempted suicide

3.5 million made suicide plans

1.4 million attempted suicide

217 thousand made no plans and attempted suicide

12 millions adults had serious thoughts of suicide

The public health approach to addressing suicide includes the entire continuum from mental health conditions, suicidal struggles and attempts, disability and morbidity related to suicide risk, and of course suicide's mortality toll.

● Suicide Loss Survivors

Additionally, suicide loss survivors comprise 30–50% of most populations with numerous individuals impacted by each suicide death.[8] The experiences of loss survivors including clinical sequelae and methods for healing through grief are important areas of research and represent opportunities for suicide postvention and prevention efforts, since 51% of a representative sample of American adults have had one or more exposures to suicide and suicide loss can increase suicide risk of those left behind.[7,9] Research is finding a host of negative health sequelae related to Complicated Grief (CG) and even more general suicide bereavement.[10,11] Health providers can become educated about the course of suicide bereavement as another critical way to provide the most effective care possible and to contribute to advances in suicide prevention. In the suicide prevention field, an undeniable truism is: "postvention is prevention," referring to the net effect of decreasing a loss survivor's own suicide risk by facilitating their healing after suicide loss, in many instances by helping to eventually empower them to become part of suicide prevention and postvention efforts. Please see Chapter 17 for more clinical tips related to the care of suicide loss survivors.

Key Point Lived Experience Perspectives
Suicide loss survivors or people bereaved by suicide loss are an important population. Not only does the loss experience represent an important part of the scope of the problem of suicide, but people bereaved by suicide can be at increased risk for suicide. Additionally, in the suicide prevention movement across several nations, suicide loss survivors were early advocates for research funding, suicide prevention education, and stigma reduction and continue to be powerful voices for change.

● Suicide: Focus on the USA

A 2018 report by the Centers for Disease Control (CDC) in the USA reveals the extent of the growing public health suicide crisis.[12] The US national rate of suicide had been decreasing from 1986 to 1999, but then unfortunately began to rise, steadily increasing each year since 1999. Increasing 1% annually from 1999 through 2006, suicides in the USA are most recently increasing by 1.5–3.7% annually. In many other western nations, suicide rates are generally decreasing, whereas in the USA the rate has been on the rise.[13] In December 2020, the CDC released 2019 national suicide data finding the US suicide rate had decreased by 2.1% year over year, the first decrease in 20 years.

CDC suicide surveillance data in the USA indicates that suicide rates are increasing for both males and females and for all age groups 10–74. It is the second leading cause of death for 15–34 year-olds, surpassed only by unintentional injuries (i.e., accidents).

For females, the increase in suicide rates was greatest and most significant in number for those between the ages of 45 and 64, and for males, also between the ages of 45 and 64. Overall, the rate for males is three to four times the rate of females (20.7 versus 5.8).

Over the past two decades, the rate of suicide in the USA has increased by 35% and is at its highest level in 30 years. Youth suicide rates in the USA are at a high point over a 40-year period, with a 2019 CDC report revealing a concerning trend among younger children and adolescents age 10–14, whose suicide rate had declined from 1.5 to 0.9 from 2000 to 2007, but has tripled from 2007 to 2017 to 2.5 per 100,000.[14]

In the USA, the most frequent suicide method used by males is firearms (55.4%), while women use poisoning most frequently (34.1%) (See Figures 14.1–14.2 and 14.3–14.4 for breakdown of suicide methods for males and females as well as for veteran males and females.) Globally, a WHO suicide mortality report finds that methods of suicide vary between countries – a difference driven primarily by availability of means.[6]

● Suicide: Focus on Asia

Of the nearly 1 million suicides globally each year, the Asian continent accounts for an estimated 60% with China, Japan, and India accounting for 40% of the world's suicides.[15] Because of religious and legal sanctions against suicide, underreporting of suicide most certainly occurs in many countries to varying degrees. Among the Asian countries where whole population suicide rates are available, South Korea has among the highest rates at 31.0/100,000 per year. Methods for suicide include the most available means, so in China, Sri Lanka, and Pakistan, where agricultural work is common, pesticides are the most common means of suicide, whereas in urban areas like Hong Kong and Singapore, jumping is the most common method. Notable suicide methods in Asia also include charcoal burning and self-immolation, which are exceedingly rare in western nations. Overall the ratio of male to female suicide rates is lower in Asian countries, closer to 2:1 (although widening over the past decade in areas like China, Taiwan, and Hong Kong) versus the 3–4:1 male to female ratio in western regions of the world. Compared with western females, Asian females tend to use more lethal means (such as pesticide poisoning, a common method among younger Chinese females), although this is changing with urbanization and suicide prevention efforts that include means restriction, regulatory changes, and education efforts focused on pesticides, targeted at both community members and pesticide vendors in Asia.

● Federal Investments in Research and Interventions Are Made for
  Other Threats to Life and Limb

Imagine the number of deaths related to a particular toxic exposure had grown
dramatically in the past 20 years. Imagine that 48,000 Americans die from this toxin
every year, making it the tenth leading cause of death in the USA, impacting all age
groups. What would be the response?

Given the $1 billion investment the US Congress made in response to the Zika
virus outbreak in 2016 to ensure that not one American would die, the several billion
dollar investment to combat the opioid crisis, and the similarly appropriately large
investment to address the Covid pandemic, one can imagine what the national
response to a toxin killing tens of thousands of Americans might be. In fact, those
approximately 50,000 deaths in the US, and more than 800,000 deaths globally, are
caused by what is indeed the tenth leading and generally preventable cause of US
mortality: suicide. Among the top ten leading causes of death pre-pandemic, suicide
is one of three that continue to be on the rise. Unfortunately, lulled by the longevity of
the problem, the shroud of stigma that has kept it in the shadows, most nations have
not launched a response commensurate with suicide's morbidity and mortality toll, and
what has clearly become a national and global crisis.

KEY TAKEAWAYS

a. As the science elucidating suicide risk and prevention continues to explode, answers are forthcoming, shedding light on suicide. It takes time for answers from science to translate into everyday knowledge about actions to take. Thus, we are currently living in a time of cultural transition when it comes to suicide prevention.

b. Find out if your country has a national suicide prevention plan and the ways that you might become more involved or serve to advance any strategies.

c. New scientific research on the clinical and community based strategies that can prevent suicide offer hope for bending the curve and reducing suicide rates.

d. Specifically research shows that 1) suicide is a generally preventable cause of death, and 2) health systems and providers have a vital role to play in suicide prevention.[16]

e. Suicide prevention and suicide prediction are concepts that tend to be conflated. Various complex health outcomes are considered preventable, without being predictable on the individual level.

f. While the drivers of suicide are complex and risk factors multiple, cultural norms in many regions of the world are changing related to mental health and suicide, with people beginning to open up and speak out about mental health, reducing the stigma around mental health, help seeking, and suicide prevention.

g. Suicide prevention can be viewed as a movement in which suicide loss survivors, people with lived experiences of attempt or suicidal struggle, and others with a personal and/or professional interest in suicide prevention are banding together, advocating for more investment in science and policy change in healthcare and beyond.

h. Surveillance of suicide attempts and deaths must improve to better measure the impact of suicide prevention efforts.

i. Suicide prevention at a broad scale includes policy changes, public health initiatives like school-based programs and universal education, health system delivery changes, and new suicide prevention focused treatments delivered in clinical settings.

j. Federal investments in suicide prevention research, community programs and clinical treatments can reduce suicide mortality.

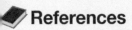

References

1 American Foundation for Suicide Prevention (n.d.) In Executive Summary: A Survey about Mental Health and Suicide in the United States. Retrieved from afsp.org/story/covid-19-reinforces-a-renewed-call-to-make-suicide-prevention-a-national-priority/.

2 American Foundation for Suicide Prevention (2018) National Survey Shows Majority of Americans Would Take Action to Prevent Suicide. afsp.org/harrispoll/.

3 World Health Organization (2013) *Mental Health Action Plan 2013–2020.* Geneva: World Health Organization.

4 World Health Organization MiNDbank www.mindbank.info/, accessed April 24, 2019. MiNDbank is an online platform for resources and national/regional level policies, strategies, laws and service standards for mental health and related areas.

5 Naghavi, M. (2019) (on behalf of the Global Burden of Disease Self-Harm Collaborators.) Global, regional, and national burden of suicide mortality 1990 to 2016: Systematic analysis for the Global Burden of Disease Study 2016. *BMJ*; 364: I94.

6 World Health Organization (2014) Preventing Suicide: A Global Imperative. Retrieved from apps.who.int/iris/bitstream/handle/10665/131056/9789241564779_eng.pdf;jsessionid=BD2F88630987953D20BB6DC50241BE19?sequence=1.

7 Cerel, J., Brown, M., Maple, M., et al. (2018) How Many People Are Exposed to Suicide? Not Six. *Suicide Life Threat Behav*, doi:10.1111/sltb.12450

8 Feigelman, W., Cerel, J., McIntosh, J., Brent, D., & Gutin, N. (2018) Suicide exposures and bereavement among American adults: Evidence from the 2016 General Social Survey. *J Affect Disord*, 227: 1–6. doi:10.1016/j.jad.2017.09.056

9 Jordan, J. R. (2017) Postvention is prevention: The case for suicide postvention, *Death Studies*, 41(10): 614–21, doi: 10.1080/07481187.2017.1335544

10 Pitman, A., Osborn, D., King, M., & Erlangsen, A. (2014) Effects of suicide bereavement on mental health and suicide risk. *Lancet Psychiatry*, 1(1): 86–94.

11 Cerel, J. & Rebecca, L. (2018) It's not who you know, it's how you think you know them: suicide exposure and suicide bereavement. *Psychoanal Study Child*, 71(1): 76–96, doi: 10.1080/00797308.2017.1415066

12 Centers for Disease Control and Prevention (2018, June 7) In "Suicide Rising Across the US". Retrieved from www.cdc.gov/vitalsigns/suicide/index.html.

13 Fond, G., Llorca, P. M., Boucekine, M., et al. (2016) Disparities in suicide mortality trends between United States of America and 25 European countries: Retrospective analysis of WHO mortality database. *Scientific Reports*, 6: 20256. doi:10.1038/srep20256

14 Curtin, S. C., & Heron, M. (2019) Death rates due to suicide and homicide among persons aged 10–24: United States, 2000–2017. NCHS Data Brief, no 352. Hyattsville, MD: National Center for Health Statistics.

15 Wu, K. C., Chen, Y. Y. & Yip, P. S. F. (2012) Suicide methods in Asia: Implications in suicide prevention. *Int. J. Environ. Res. Public Health*, 9: 1135–58.

16 Mann J.J., Michel C.A., Auerbach R.P. (2021) Improving suicide prevention through evidence-based strategies: A systematic review. *Am J Psychiatry*, doi:10.1176/appi.ajp.2020.20060864

2

Dispelling Myths Surrounding Suicide

11 Myth-Busting Truths

1. People who take their lives are not necessarily weak or cowardly.

2. Suicide is multifactorial and not caused by any single event, stressor, or risk factor.

3. Risk is highly dynamic, not set in stone.

4. The majority of people who survive suicide attempts go on to live and thrive.

5. Suicidal "gestures" are actually meaningful indicators of risk, a way of communicating need for help.

6. People who talk about suicidal thoughts are revealing true potential suicide risk.

7. The experience of losing someone to suicide feels sudden, like being blindsided. This does not mean that suicide lacks an actual build up.

8. When lethal means are less accessible, suicide risk is greatly diminished.

9. Just one person can make a difference. Each of us has the ability to help tilt the balance for someone toward hope and survival.

10. By having a caring conversation and asking about suicidal thoughts, the at-risk individual has more opportunity to share, connect, and receive support.

11. Suicide is not as simple as a "rational choice."

Introduction

For many complex health issues throughout history, misinformed views tend to promulgate, leading to a multitude of negative effects, deeply stigmatizing the experiences where these health issues are involved. Without science, untruths and stigma continue to thrive. In the past, before a body of scientific research led to an understanding of what drives suicide risk, many myths prevailed about suicide. These myths not only shaped stigmatized and erroneous views of suicidal behavior but resulted in harshly punitive ideas and judgment of people who experience suicidal thoughts, who attempt, or who ultimately lose their lives to suicide. Now that a multi-disciplinary group of scientific fields is shedding tremendous light on the actual drivers of suicide risk, cultural views are changing, bringing an understanding that while complex, suicide is a health issue.

One myth that may still have echoes in the current day is the erroneous idea that certain individuals are "bent" on suicide, and therefore very little can be done to change course once someone becomes suicidal. Today, scientific research in a broad range of domains – from neuroscience to clinical research to epidemiology and community/public health interventions – shows that despite its complexity, suicide is 1) a health-related outcome and 2) largely preventable.

To understand how suicide can, in many instances, be prevented, and the role health professionals can play in preventing suicide, it is first important to dispel the myths that lead to erroneous assumptions about suicidal behavior and suicide. This chapter sets out 11 truths with their corollary myths about suicide. These myths must be dispelled so that they may no longer undermine efforts to prevent suicide.

 Key Points

- Science is shedding light and busting the myths that long prevailed about suicide.

- These myths not only shaped stigmatized and incorrect views of suicidal behavior, but resulted in incorrect, punitive, judgmental ideas about people who struggle with suicidal thoughts, attempts, or who ultimately go on to lose their lives to suicide.

- Now that several scientific fields are shedding tremendous light on the actual drivers of suicide risk, cultural views are changing, understanding that while complex, suicide is a health issue.

B | PRINCIPLES

- Science of suicide risk and prevention is growing at a strong pace.

- The findings from research are shedding light on ways we can understand and prevent suicide.

- Prevailing myths are still prevalent since the translation and dissemination from scientific discovery to cultural beliefs and universal knowledge takes time and effort.

- Some of the most prevalent and harmful myths are addressed in this chapter with their corollary "truth" presented first.

- For example, suicide should not be thought of in terms of weakness or cowardice. Just as those who die from other health outcomes after a "strong fight" with their illness are not considered weak, the same holds true for people who die by suicide.

- While suicide can be precipitated by a triggering event, suicide is not thought to be caused by one factor or event. Psychological autopsy method research clearly demonstrates there are multiple risk factors that converge or escalate at a moment of acute risk. While we do not always recognize all of the risk factors clearly at the time, suicide risk usually builds over time with changes in health – brain and body, cognition, perception, sense of hope, social connection.

- Because stigma is pervasive and human instinct is to withdraw and isolate when suffering, many hide distressing internal experiences, making suicide seem "out of the blue", but it is not usually the case. Even in more impulsive cases of suicidal behavior, there are usually numerous other longer term risk factors at play.

- Suicidal people are not usually "bent on suicide" but rather are more often ambivalent and can often readily move closer to their reasons for living and sense of hope.

- It is not the case that a history of attempting suicide indicates the person is destined to attempt again or die by suicide. In fact, more than 90% of people who live through an even medically serious suicide attempt do not go on to die by suicide.

- Our clinical lens can be shaped by understanding that "manipulation" is not at the root of most suicidal behavior (although some clinical settings do select for more secondary gain behaviors). A "cry for help" is just that: a signal of distress that warrants intervention for an at-risk individual.

- It is not the case that people who express suicidal thoughts are less at risk or simply talking rather than acting. Many who die by suicide had spoken of taking their life, sometimes directly and sometimes indirectly.

- It is not the case that suicidal people will simply find another method if their identified method is not readily accessible.

- Asking a patient directly and compassionately if they are thinking about ending their life is a safe and effective way to approach the issue. It is a myth that raising the question will increase risk or "plant the idea" in a person's mind.

- Suicide risk is multi-faceted, dynamic, and often builds over time, therefore there are many opportunities for intervention and prevention.

C Myth-Busting Truths about Suicide

1 People who take their lives are not weak or cowardly

The old idea about people who take their lives being weak or cowardly stems from ignorance about what drives suicide risk. Health factors related to suicide include mental health and physical health conditions, brain structure and functioning, genetics, psychological make-up, and life stressors. Many factors contribute to the path to suicide, and therefore extremely strong people have taken their lives – having nothing to do with fortitude of character, but because they are human – and these risk factors exist and impact all human beings. People who die by suicide have often fought long and hard to survive and live through extreme levels of mental anguish and/ or physical pain. The very construct of weakness or cowardice does not fit for suicide in the same way as it has no place in considering why people die of cancer or any other health-related outcome. Patients can die from other health outcomes after a "strong fight" with their illness, and the same holds true for people who die by suicide.

> *Those who die from other health outcomes after a "strong fight" with their illness are not considered weak, and the same holds true for people who die by suicide.*

2 Suicide is multifactorial and not a one-cause-effect phenomenon

While external stressors are the most visible to outside observers and the media, science has clearly shown there are always multiple risk factors that contribute to suicide. Risk factors including mental health conditions (such as depression or major depressive disorder (MDD), substance use problems, bipolar disorder, borderline personality disorder, schizophrenia, post traumatic stress disorder (PTSD), other anxiety disorders, and eating disorders) are among the most common and forceful risk factors for suicide.[1] Additionally brain and cognitive changes occur during periods of suicide risk, such as a constriction of cognition: coping strategies become temporarily less accessible to people who find themselves in a state of tunnel vision.[2] For people at increased risk for suicide, studies have shown that their brains may have a more profound stress response.[3]

> *Suicide is not caused by any one event or factor.*

3 Suicide risk is highly dynamic, not set in stone

Suicide risk is extremely dynamic. For people at risk of suicide, their risk can change day by day and even hour to hour. The idea that suicidal people are "bent on it" is completely erroneous in most instances. Suicidal ideation and planning come from the human mind's strong need to problem-solve a solution to pain, despair, and hopelessness. But the human spirit of survival and resilience, of wanting to find hope, is also strongly at play. Therefore, ambivalence is part of the suicidal process. And intense periods of high suicide risk are actually relatively short, often lasting minutes to hours. As a result, providing someone with support and keeping them safe during a high intensity period of risk is most often lifesaving.

> *Suicidal people usually are not "bent on suicide" but rather are ambivalent and can find hope and recovery. There are many opportunities for intervention and prevention.*

4 The majority of people who survive nearly lethal attempts go on to live and thrive

People who attempt suicide have revealed through their ability to move from ideation to attempt behavior, that they have a potentially higher lifetime risk of suicide. Thus, a past attempt is one of the strongest predictors of future suicidal behavior. That said, the vast majority who survive an attempt do NOT go on to take their lives. The vast majority (85-95%) of those who survive a suicide attempt go on to live out a natural lifespan.[4]

> *It is not the case that a history of attempt suicide indicates the person is destined to attempt again or die by suicide.*

5 Suicidal "gestures" are actually meaningful indicators of risk, a way of communicating need for help

The dichotomous construct that people are either "just being manipulative" or have "serious risk" does not fit with suicide. It is erroneous and actually dangerous thinking to only hold this black-or-white view of suicidal behavior. Self-injurious actions with any intent of dying are signs of distress that warrant action. Since suicidal behavior stems from a wide array of psychopathology, genetic, and environmental influences, some behaviors may be more chronic and repetitive, while others seem out of character, appearing to come "out of the blue." But in all cases, research has shown that people who attempt suicide, and people with a history of nonsuicidal self-injury, have an elevated risk for suicide over the long term. The treatment plan for each individual case is different and should ideally be tailored to the most powerful drivers of that individual's suicidal behavior. Also the fact that people who attempt suicide always have a mixture of ambivalence, a certain ratio of survival instinct and desire to live, alongside some level of intent to die in order to escape pain, does not change the health risk these behaviors indicate. In these ways, a "cry for help" is truly an important and useful expression of need for support and treatment.

> A "cry for help" is just that: a signal of distress that warrants intervention for an at-risk individual. Be wary of assumptions about manipulation or which equate chronic behavior patterns with lack of risk.

6 People who talk about suicidal thoughts are revealing true potential suicide risk

More than 50% of people who take their lives talk with a family member, friend, or healthcare provider about suicide within the weeks before their death.[5] Some have incorrectly thought that "the people who talk about their suicidal thoughts are not the ones to worry about." There is simply no correlation between how people do or do not express their distress and their true level of suicide risk. Many factors lead people to hide their distress, but some people are more able to disclose their feelings for a variety of reasons. Even people who try to keep their distress private will often give some verbal clues regarding their frame of mind, sometimes expressed through jokes or other oblique statements.

> It is not the case that people who express suicidal thoughts are less at risk or simply talking rather than acting. Most people who died by suicide had spoken of taking their life, sometimes directly and sometimes indirectly.

Case Example: Truth/Myth #6

The beloved celebrity chef and travel documentarian, Anthony Bourdain, tragically died by suicide in 2018. While the world felt blindsided and viewers of his show "Parts Unknown," friends, colleagues, and fans were shocked by his death, the truth is that he had mentioned his despair and/or suicidal thoughts over 15 times on air or in public interviews. Over several years, he repeatedly mentioned the idea of taking his life by the specific method he eventually did use to take his life, even including the location of his "lonely hotel room." No one knew to take him seriously at the time and likely thought he was being facetious, fitting with his often sarcastic, sharp witted humor. We are often lulled into thinking that people with a record of successful achievements or intermittent joie de vivre are somehow protected from suicide risk. Although much clearer in hindsight, we are all learning to pay attention to statements that either directly or indirectly provide a window into an individual's suffering or actual suicidal thoughts.

7 The experience of losing someone to suicide feels sudden, like you've been blindsided. This does not mean that suicide lacks an actual build up

It is understandable that we do not always see warning signs and risk factors plainly. In the majority of suicide cases, in retrospect it becomes clearer that the person showed signs of suicide risk from changes in behavior, mood, sleep, substance use, to talking in different ways from their typical ways – about being overwhelmed, hopeless, or like a burden. As a society we are learning to connect the dots of these warning signs with life stressors or health changes and learn what to do, especially as healthcare providers. It is critical to understand that people who are in psychological pain often do not express their internal experiences overtly for several reasons including stigma and cultures emphasizing self-sufficiency, and they often put feelers out to determine who is a safe person to disclose their suicidal ideation to. Be sure to approach people you care about who are struggling with a clear message of respect, love, and compassion; tell them you will not judge them for any challenge they are facing.

> *While we understandably cannot see all of the risk factors clearly at the time, suicide risk usually builds over time with changes in health – brain and body, cognition, perception, sense of hope, social connection. Because stigma is pervasive and human instinct is to withdraw and isolate when suffering, many hide these internal experiences, making suicide seem "out of the blue" but it is not usually the case. Suicides are not generally purely impulsive without other risk factors.*

8 When lethal means are less accessible, suicide risk is greatly diminished

A body of research on various forms of lethal means studied including bridges, pesticides, carbon monoxide, and firearms, consistently tell the same story: when you make commonly used lethal means for a population less accessible, the rate of suicide for the entire population decreases, even when other means are available. Additionally other research shows that while switching to a different suicide method can occur, it actually occurs less than 35–40% of the time.[6]

> *It is not the case that if you make a person's suicide method inaccessible, it will not make a difference because suicidal people will find another method.*

9 Just one person can make a difference. You have the ability to help tilt the balance for someone toward hope and survival

Humans are social creatures and have a basic need to feel connected to others, to family, and community. So even though in western society, people may be viewed as autonomous and independent, the truth is that we are extremely social beings with a basic need for connection. Experiencing the caring concern of others, or even (sometimes very appropriately) the paternalistic treatment/guidance given by health providers, family members, or close friends especially during a health crisis, helps us tremendously, changing the way we experience ourselves in the world and positively impacting our mental and physical health.

> *It is not the case that we are helpless or unable to support and potentially influence a suicidal patient or loved one. Providing a sense of connection or support can save a life.*

10 By having a caring conversation and asking about suicidal thoughts, you are providing support

Studies and clinical experience find that people feel a sense of relief when asked about how deeply their pain is affecting them, including asking about suicidal thoughts. People are not harmed by being asked about suicide whether they are having thoughts of suicide or not, especially when asked in a caring, non-judgmental way.[7]

> *It is not the case that you should refrain from asking if someone is suicidal because you could plant the idea or make them worse.*

11 Suicide is not as simple as a "rational" choice

A growing body of neuroscience research finds that temporary, almost always very transient, brain changes occur during periods of suicidal crisis.[2] So while there may be very rare circumstances when a person chooses to take their life without their cognition being significantly influenced by mental illness or other health factors (such as extreme mental anguish, pain, psychosis, hopelessness, or desperation) the vast majority of suicide attempts and death by suicide are not choices the person would have made in their usual cognitive state when they routinely used a variety of coping strategies to deal with challenges.

> *While there may be rare instances of ending one's life related to factors other than these, science demonstrates that health factors and brain changes during suicidal crisis create cognitive constriction and a temporary but significant inability to access usual coping strategies.*

Key Point

Suicide Risk Is Multi-Faceted and There Are Many Opportunities for Prevention

As the myths above indicate, there was a time when suicide was considered the result of a fluke moment in time in which a person suddenly, impulsively "lost their head" and took their life. An alternative explanation for a suicide was that the person was chronically weak in the areas of character, problem-solving ability, or fortitude, and had simply been overcome by life's challenges.

Not only untrue, these myths related to character and strength, judging and keeping people who suffer living in silence. They are inconsistent with a large body of research that demonstrates that suicide is a complex health outcome.

- When suicide risk escalates, it is driven by multiple risk factors, albeit often undetected during life.

- Suicide is multifactorial. Research clearly shows that mental health conditions, genetic and other neurobiological factors, cultural, perceived, or systemic barriers to effective treatment for depression and other mental illness, sense of isolation or rejection versus support and connection, past traumatic events versus resilience building influences, accessibility of lethal means in the home or community, and cultural beliefs about mental health and suicide, all play significant roles in a population's and a person's risk for suicide.

- Science has shed light on the risk factors for suicide, as well as the protective factors that make suicide a less likely outcome for individuals. Identifying the risk factors, protective factors, and warning signs as early as possible is the foundation of saving a life to suicide.

- We now know that preventing suicide can occur along a long upstream continuum: a potentially lethal attempt can be averted at the moment of suicidal crisis, but also earlier intervention that prevents or mitigates the impact of risk factors such as early childhood trauma, adverse events, abuse, exposure to others' suicides, etc. can also prevent loss of life to suicide much later.

KEY TAKEAWAYS

a. Those who die from other health outcomes after a "strong fight" with their illness are not considered weak, and the same holds true for people who die by suicide.

b. Research demonstrates that suicide is not generally caused by any one event or factor.

c. Suicidal people are not usually "bent on suicide" but rather are ambivalent and can often readily find hope and recovery.

d. It is not the case that a history of attempted suicide indicates the person is destined to attempt again or die by suicide.

e. A "cry for help" is just that: a signal of distress that warrants intervention for an at-risk individual.

f. It is not the case that people who express suicidal thoughts are less at risk or are simply talking rather than acting. Many who die by suicide had spoken of taking their life, sometimes directly and sometimes indirectly.

g. While we cannot always see risk factors clearly, suicide risk usually builds over time with changes in health – brain and body, cognition, perception, sense of hope, social connection.

h. Because stigma is pervasive and human instinct is to withdraw and isolate when distress sets in, many hide their suffering and internal experiences, making suicide seem "out of the blue" or impulsive, but that is most often not the case.

i. Suicides are not generally purely impulsive without other risk factors.

j. It is not the case that if you make a person's suicide method inaccessible, it will not make a difference because suicidal people will find another method. While some do substitute method, with the brief element of time introduced, the majority shift back into normal cognitive thought processes with other coping options available to them again.

k. It is not the case that you should not ask if someone is suicidal because you could plant the idea or make them worse. Through a caring, non-judgmental approach, research shows the suicidal person usually feels a sense of connection and hope by sharing their experiences and receiving support.

l. Suicide is not as simple as a "rational choice."

m. Suicide risk is multi-faceted, dynamic, and often builds over time, therefore there are many opportunities for intervention and prevention.

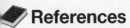

References

1   Cavanagh, J. T. O., Carson, A. J., Sharpe, M., & Lawrie, S. M. (2003) Psychological autopsy studies of suicide: A systematic review. *Psychol Med*, 33(3): 395–405.

2   Dombrovski, A. Y., & Hallquist, M. N. (2017) The decision neuroscience perspective on suicidal behavior: Evidence and hypotheses. *Curr Opin Psychiatry*, 30(1): 7–14.

3   Oquendo, M. A., Sullivan, G. M., Sudol, K., et al. (2014) Toward a biosignature for suicide. *American J Psychiatry*, 171(12): 1259–77.

4   Hawton, K., Zahl, D., & Weatherall, R. (2003) Suicide following deliberate self-harm: Long-term follow-up of patients who presented to a general hospital. *Br Psychiatry*, 182(6): 537–42.

5   Pompili, M., Belvederi Murri, M., Patti, S., et al. (2016) The communication of suicidal intentions: A meta-analysis. *Psychol Med*, 46(11): 2239–53. doi:10.1017/S0033291716000696

6   Gunnell, D., & Miller, M. (2010) Strategies to prevent suicide. *BMJ*, 341: 157–58.

7   Gould, M. S., Marrocco, F. A., Kleinman, M., et al. (2005) Evaluating iatrogenic risk of youth suicide screening programs: A randomized controlled trial. *JAMA*, 293(13): 1635–43. doi:10.1001/jama.293.13.1635

3

The Public Health Model of Suicide Prevention

QUICK CHECK

 ### A   Introduction

The science of suicide risk and prevention is growing, making one thing very clear. While suicide risk involves a complex set of risk factors, the end common pathway is a life-threatening health crisis. As is the case with all health-related causes of death, a robust public health strategy can reduce mortality. This chapter provides a framework for understanding the public health approach to preventing suicide. Examples of effective public health suicide prevention strategies at national and regional levels are provided.

B   PRINCIPLES

- As is the case with all complex health problems, a robust public health strategy can reduce suicide mortality.

- The public health model is a multi-tiered approach including universal education and health promotion, selective and targeted prevention, and treatment and recovery.

- Successful suicide prevention programs have been carried out at the national level as well as at local community levels.

- Examples of suicide prevention efforts that have reduced suicide rates include a program in New Mexico focused on American Indian youth, a US Air Force Program, a province-wide program in Québec, a classroom management program for kindergarteners and first graders, and the Garrett Lee Smith Memorial Grants in the USA.

- National suicide prevention programs with full scale implementation that have proven successful include those in Finland, Norway, Sweden, and Australia.

- In addition to community level prevention, healthcare settings have a critical role to play in preventing suicide. This includes behavioral healthcare, primary care, and all healthcare settings.

- Language related to suicide is important, to be in line with science-informed ideas, to correct myths, and to be respectful of people with lived experience and/or loss. Language tips are provided.

C The Public Health Approach to Suicide Prevention

Figure 3.1 Public health approach

Optimal results are achieved with a multi-layered approach to achieve health outcome goals, including suicide prevention. When health promotion and prevention tactics at all levels are strategic and sustained, and when treatment and recovery resources are well developed and accessible to the population, the opportunity to reduce suicide mortality is optimized.[1]

National Collaborating Centre for Mental Health (UK). Antenatal and Postnatal Mental Health: Clinical Management and Service Guidance: Updated edition. Leicester (UK): British Psychological Society; 2014 Dec. (NICE Clinical Guidelines, No. 192.) Figure 1 [The mental health intervention spectrum]. Available from: www.ncbi.nlm.nih.gov/books/NBK338542/figure/app9.f1/

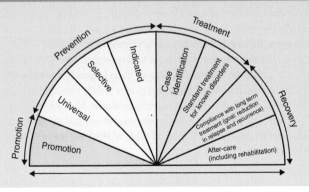

Why Universal Education Matters for Suicide Prevention

When community members share a basic common knowledge about a health issue, stigma is reduced and family members, schools, and workplaces are able to apply that knowledge to their daily lives and work in several ways: to build healthier families and communities, to recognize risk when present, and to lead at-risk individuals to seek medical/professional evaluation and treatment.

Examples of Mental Health Education Campaigns

Health promotion for suicide prevention includes pro mental health ad campaigns such as SeizeTheAwkward (developed by the Ad Council, the American Foundation for Suicide Prevention (AFSP), and the Jed Foundation), #RealConvo (AFSP), and #BeThe1To (Lifeline), which teach basic principles of the importance of communicating about mental health needs both for oneself and with others.

Prevention strategies can target three levels for suicide prevention: **universal** (e.g., resilience and mental health promotion, safe media messaging, lethal means reduction, increased access to support/mental health services), **selective** (e.g., screening programs, training for specific roles who work with subsets of the population – teachers, corrections professionals, health providers), and **indicated** (e.g., intervention for those whose risk is detected, case management, skills training for high risk groups).

You as a health professional have a role to play in preventing suicide at all spokes of the wheel of prevention and intervention. By speaking out, **educating** patients and families about mental health and suicide **prevention**, you are serving as an effective mental health educator/promoter. By screening patients for mental health and suicide risk or facilitating a support group for at-risk LGBTQ youth, you are doing **selective prevention**. When you treat patients for depression, anxiety, PTSD, eating disorders, and addiction, you are doing **targeted prevention**. And when you hone in on suicidal thoughts and provide specific care steps outlined in Chapters 6–8, you are providing risk reducing **treatment**. When you follow up with patients and continue to check in and provide support, and help the family know how to provide support after a suicidal crisis has resolved, you are participating in patients' **recovery**.

D **Examples of Universal Prevention through Programs in Schools and Communities**

Implementing key strategies across an entire population (universal) can drive down suicide rates.[1] Suicide prevention efforts are therefore critically important at regional and national levels. In addition to effective healthcare showing evidence for reducing suicide risk, other types of interventions at the community level have found promising results for reducing suicide risk.

Examples of Effective Risk Reducing Community Based Programs

- **Model Adolescent Suicide Prevention Program for American Indian Youth in New Mexico**: reduced the number of adolescent suicide attempts by an astonishing 80% between 1988 and 2002, using lay education, trained peers, and referral to counseling.[2] Psychiatric conditions often have their onset early in the life cycle, with 50% of all mental illness manifesting prior to age 14. So identifying mental health conditions in children and adolescents and ensuring that effective and ongoing treatment is provided, or ways to reduce the morbidity and mortality, are examples of a critical approach to reducing the morbidity and mortality associated with mental illness, including preventing suicide risk in youth or later life.

- **Sources of Strength** shifted schoolwide coping and help seeking norms and improved students' perceptions of adult availability using student "peer leaders" to deliver messaging and conduct prevention activities to enhance healthy coping and help seeking norms.[3]

- **Wingman-Connect: US Air Force.**[4] A universal intervention that focuses on building protective factors among classes of young enlisted personnel was rigorously evaluated in technical training school. Airmen in Wingman-Connect trained classes reported significantly lower suicide and depression scale scores one month after training, and after six months the likelihood of a trainee reporting elevated risk for suicidal thoughts and behaviors was 19% lower, just outside of conventional statistical significance (p = .067). Wingman-Connect is, to our knowledge, the first prevention training evaluated through a randomized controlled trial (RCT) that reduced risk for suicidal thoughts/behaviors and depression in a general Air Force population.

- A trend analysis in the **US Air Force Suicide Prevention Program** showed that suicide rates of Air Force members decreased by 33% between 1996 and 2004 while a comprehensive program was enacted to educate all levels of the force on warning signs and help seeking. Rates in the US population were also decreasing during that time, so it is not clear that the change was due to the program but the results were encouraging.[5]

- **Help for Life Program, Québec, Canada**: A multi-pronged approach involving 40 organizations in Québec to carry out a province-wide prevention strategy, including media, training, and youth referrals to mental healthcare; 33% reduction in province suicide rate from 1999 to 2012.[6]

- **The Good Behavior Game**: a universal classroom behavior management method, tested in first- and second-grade classrooms in inner city Baltimore, Maryland beginning in the 1985–1986 school year. Follow-up at ages 19–21 found significantly lower rates of drug and alcohol use disorders, regular smoking, antisocial personality disorder, delinquency, and incarceration for violent crimes, and >50% less prevalence of suicidal ideation among students who had been in classes using the Good Behavior Game method.[7]

Figure 3.2 Examples of effective national rate reductions

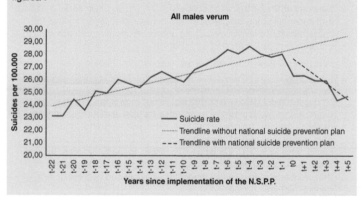

Trends in male suicide rates in four nations with national suicide prevention plans implemented and sustained over five years versus males in four control countries without a national prevention plan.

https://bmcpsychiatry.biomedcentral.com/articles/10.1186/s12888-019-2147-y/figures/1

Examples of National Suicide Prevention Programs that reduced rates

A study of four countries (Finland, Norway, Sweden, and Australia) with full scale implementation of national suicide prevention plans compared the trends in suicide rates over the years before and after plan launch, with four control countries without such plans (Canada, Austria, Switzerland, and Denmark), matched for factors such as culture, religion, population, and surveillance of suicide rates. This analysis found a reduction in suicide rates especially among the adult male populations of the countries with suicide prevention plans compared with the countries without plans.[8] Strategies in suicide prevention plans for these nations include a public health approach utilizing universal education about mental health, suicide risk factors, and warning signs, and resources for support, crisis level support, and mental healthcare. Additionally efforts to optimize engagement of high risk populations, shore up crisis services, and enhance suicide prevention within healthcare settings with a focus on screening and continuity across transitions of care are common approaches.

 Youth Suicide Prevention Advocacy Initiative that Reduced Rates

● Evidence for Suicide Reduction with Universal and Selective Prevention

Another powerful example of evidence for the effectiveness of universal and selective suicide prevention programming is the Garrett Lee Smith (GLS) Memorial Act grant, which has funded youth suicide prevention activities in the USA since 2004 on college campus, community, and tribal settings in many states. Over a 15-year period, a large portion of counties in the USA received financial support to engage in youth suicide prevention initiatives including outreach, awareness raising, screening, "gatekeeper" training (meaning training for key front-line roles to recognize risk and act), developing coalitions, policies/protocols, and supporting crisis support hotlines. A total of 40% of GLS grants are awarded in rural areas of the USA where suicide rates are higher and where resources for programs and clinical treatment tend to be much lower. In a major evaluation study, counties with GLS activities were compared with control counties unexposed to GLS programs (matched for demographic characteristics, race/ethnicity make-up, median household income, unemployment rates, and suicide rates of youth and adults), and significant reductions were found both for short- and longer-term impact on suicidal behaviors and suicide deaths. The positive effect was greatest in rural areas of the USA.[9]

 Healthcare Settings: Focus on Primary Care

These striking examples of suicide prevention programs at the community level reveal the potential to prevent suicide through concentrated efforts based on training and programs in non-clinical settings, informed by the latest research and knowledge. The greatest evidence for the potential to save lives, however, is in the clinical arena. Science has provided particular clinical interventions developed with suicide risk reduction in mind. These treatments and simple steps for identifying risk and providing basic care steps and communication reduce suicide risk.

Key Point. The best evidence in the suicide prevention science points to the clinical arena, where populations who are at risk of suicide present for healthcare, and where detecting those at risk and providing evidence-based strategies and treatments can save many lives.

● Focus on Primary Care

There are many reasons health settings represent the best hope for lifesaving intervention.

Primary care, behavioral health, emergency care – all healthcare settings – are critical to the mission of suicide prevention: we all have a role to save lives. Behavioral health settings have long been considered the main setting where suicide preventive care is delivered. And it is certainly true that psychiatric patient populations generally carry higher risk for suicide. All patients with psychiatric conditions should be routinely and regularly screened and assessed for suicide risk. Treatment and closer follow-up care in behavioral health is indeed a key strategy to decrease risk and address suffering in high risk patient populations. Several medications and specialized forms of psychotherapy have been shown to reduce suicidal behavior; these specialized treatments are usually delivered in behavioral health settings. (See Chapters 7 and 9 for more on suicide preventive treatments.)

However, primary care providers treat all of these same patients and more. Primary care providers also use antidepressants and other psychotropic medications, and when used judiciously, can in fact reduce suicide risk.[10] Thus, suicide prevention should be occurring across all types of health settings, including primary care and other tertiary medical and surgical settings – it can be scaled in this way to optimize all people's access to suicide risk reducing care. This could at least partially address problems with health disparities if any point of contact with a health system imparted suicide prevention-savvy care.

Settings: Primary Care

There are several reasons primary care plays a critical role in suicide prevention, in addition to behavioral health specialists.

1. **Primary care can routinely screen for and identify the emergence of or worsening in mental health problems.** While every instance of suicide has many causes, 85%–95% of the people who died by suicide were suffering from a diagnosable mental illness, albeit often unrecognized, untreated, or undertreated.[11] Among the mental health

conditions that increase risk for suicide, major depression is the most highly prevalent, present in approximately 50–60% of cases of suicide, and potent as a driver of cognitive distortion, pain, and hopelessness in many cases. However, there is a shortage and distribution problem of the workforce necessary to provide mental healthcare to the population. Additionally, even in areas where mental healthcare providers abound, many people prefer to have their mood and anxiety concerns addressed by their primary care provider, either because they know and trust their provider or are accustomed to bringing new concerns up in the primary care setting, people often attribute symptoms to physical non-psychiatric conditions, or they may simply be hesitant to seek care in an unfamiliar setting or one that feels stigmatizing to them.

2. **Primary care is poised to detect and address potential changes in suicide risk.** One study showed that from 18% to as many as 40% of people who died by suicide visited their primary care physicians within one week prior to their death.[12] Some of these visits were suicide or mental health related, many were not overt, but they all represent opportunities to uncover burgeoning risk and to act in simple ways to reduce risk (which are covered in Chapters 5–8). Additionally, as noted above, many patients prefer to have their mental health needs addressed by their primary care provider whom they may have known over long periods of time. Moreover, vigilant care of depression in primary care settings has been shown to reduce the suicide rate for that patient population.[13]

3. **Twice as many patients who die by suicide visit their primary care physicians versus a mental health professional.** One study showed that 45% of individuals dying by suicide visited their primary care physician in the month before their death. Only 20% saw a mental health professional in the same time period. This study also noted that women and older patients were more likely to have seen a mental health professional during that period.[14] Primary care is simply more accessible and normalized for many people to receive care of all kinds.

4. **Changes in physical health, the overt targets of primary care, can signal suicide risk.** Risk factors for suicide include physical health conditions such as chronic pain, trauma/brain injury, common chronic medical problems, and new or deteriorating health problems. When patients receive a new serious diagnosis, and when physical health problems are comorbid with depression or other mental health conditions, suicide risk increases can be detected.

For all of these reasons, mental health concerns are being detected and treated in primary care, at a wider scale from a public health perspective, than in behavioral health settings. Increasingly, mental health is viewed as an integral part of human health, and as one of the components of health that warrants screening at a minimum and in many cases care and ongoing maintenance, in the primary care setting. Primary care professionals, including internists and family physicians, write most of the antidepressant prescriptions – more than 60% according to one study.[15] Of pediatricians who were queried about their likelihood to treat a teenage patient with depression with an antidepressant versus refer to a child psychiatrist, only a third said they would feel comfortable treating moderate depression and one quarter severe depression. In contrast, pediatricians were five times more likely to recommend or prescribe an antidepressant if they had access to an onsite or local mental health professional.[16]

In 2018, the American Academy of Pediatrics updated their guidelines for identifying and treating childhood and teen depression, other mental health problems, and suicide risk, recognizing that pediatricians and other primary care providers are often in the best position to identify and help struggling children and teens.[17]

A study involving three pediatric clinics showed that a brief standardized screening for suicide risk in pediatric primary care practices increased detection rates of suicidal youth by nearly 400% and increased referrals to outpatient behavioral care centers by the same rate.[18]

Primary Care Example: Reducing Suicide – The Hungary Study

In a five-year, AFSP-funded study that trained primary care physicians to diagnose and treat depression in a region of Hungary with one of the highest suicide rates in the world, the potential for suicide prevention was demonstrated.

Over the past 100 years, Hungary has been among the nations with the highest average suicide rate, and within Hungary, the county with one of the highest suicide rates is Bacs-Kiskun. The study involved two regions in Bacs-Kiskun: Kiskunhalas region, which is where the suicide prevention intervention occurred; and nearby Kiskunfelegyhaza region, which was the control region. The two regions share similar suicide rates, similar demographic characteristics (for example, both regions had more than 50% women and nearly a quarter of individuals who were 60 years or older), and the same emphasis on agriculture as a major source of livelihood. The intervention region was more populated than the control region (73,000 people compared to 54,000 people) but the majority lived in small villages and on farms; two-thirds of the population in the control region lived in the region's largest town.

A total of 28 of the 30 primary care providers agreed to participate in the project. The opening training session, in the form of a lecture, covered a range of suicide-related topics, from the epidemiology, recognition, and treatment of depression to a discussion on the suicide problem in the region, and from the primary care provider's role in preventing suicide to training in suicide risk recognition and appropriate responses. While the original training was lecture-based, follow-up "booster" sessions were interactive, with emphasis on Q&A, as well as case studies of recent suicides. In addition, three times per year for each of the five years, the primary care providers and their nurses were invited to lectures on suicide prevention topics.

At the end of the study period, the research team analyzed the two regions' suicide rates – the primary outcome – and antidepressant prescription rates. The suicide rate in the intervention region declined from 59.7 to 49.9 per 100,000 inhabitants, a significant decrease compared to the other counties in the region and compared to the country as a whole. Female suicides in rural areas decreased by 34% in the intervention region, while increasing by 90% in the control region. Concerning the secondary outcome, treatment for depression increased in the intervention region compared to the control region, the county, and the country.

In sum, the intervention led to a significant decline in suicide rates compared to the control county and the nation as a whole and an increase in the treatment for depression. The conclusion is clear: training of primary care physicians can make a difference in suicide rates – even in a region with one of the highest suicide rates in the world.[11]

Thus, when we say suicide is a preventable cause of death, we mean that, like other health-related mortality, investments in research and a sustained, strategic public health approach reduce mortality, but do not necessarily drive mortality to zero. The good news is that science is providing clear strategies for prevention and intervention, and it is time to translate that science into practice.

H | **Language Tips and Definitions**

Advances in science, advocacy, and stigma reduction have led to an evolution in terminology. Recommendations are provided below regarding the terms to understand and use (blue box), to use with caution to avert unintended implications (yellow box), and to avoid (pink box).

● Language and Definitions Related to Suicide

Terms to Use: Definitions

Below are the terms, with their definitions, that are considered current:

o **Suicide:** Death caused by self-directed injurious behavior with any intent to die as a result of the behavior.

o **Suicidal behavior:** Encompasses a spectrum of behavior from suicide attempt and preparatory behaviors to completed suicide.

o **Suicide attempt:** A non-fatal self-directed potentially injurious behavior with any intent to die as a result of the behavior.

o **Suicidal ideation:** Thinking about, considering, or planning suicide.

o **Suicide loss survivor** or **suicide bereaved:** Family members, friends, or colleagues of a person who died by suicide.

o **People with lived experience (of suicide), attempt survivors:** A term for people with their own personal experience with suicidal thoughts or attempt(s). An important group in the advocacy movement of suicide prevention, joining with loss survivors and other advocates.

o **Died by suicide:** This is recommended language and has replaced the phrase "committed suicide" as the preferred term. Other plain language is acceptable as well, e.g., "killed himself," "ended her life," "took their life."

● Terminology Tips

Terms to Use with Caution Related to Clarity

The following terms warrant clarification:

o **Non-suicidal self-injury (NSSI) and self-injurious behavior (SIB):** NSSI and SIB are defined as deliberately injuring oneself without suicidal intent. The most common form of NSSI is self-cutting, but other forms include burning, scratching, hitting, intentionally preventing wounds from healing, and other similar behaviors. While the behavior itself is without suicidal intent, people who have a pattern of NSSI have been found to have a higher risk of suicide in the long term.

o **Suicidality:** While this term is used frequently in clinical settings between professionals to mean the spectrum of possible suicidal experiences, it does not specify ideation, attempt, chronic/recurrent or singular event. In many instances, communication can be more effective and clear if one articulates the actual issue at hand, such as ideation or attempt, and includes any relevant details.

● Terms to Avoid Related to Suicide

Terms to Avoid

The following are current terminology recommendations:

o The phrase "commit suicide" is no longer recommended because it stems from a time when suicide was considered a criminal or morally reprehensible act. Now that science sheds light on the health issues that drive suicide risk, this term is no longer appropriate, perpetuates stigma, and is in fact no longer recommended by the *Associated Press Stylebook* (2015). Preferred language includes "died by suicide," "ended his/her life," or "killed him/herself."

o The terms "gesture" and "manipulative" imply that the behavior does not warrant serious concern. Actually, any suicidal thinking or behavior should be interpreted as a way of expressing a deep level of distress that warrants a serious, albeit customized, response.

o "Failed attempt" and "successful attempt" are simply unnecessary since the term "attempt" implies that the person did not die. And these words also carry an overtone of judgment, which should be avoided when addressing any serious health concern.

KEY TAKEAWAYS

a. As is true for all complex health outcomes, a robust public health strategy can reduce suicide mortality.

b. The public health model includes a layered approach with universal education and health promotion, selective and targeted prevention, treatment and recovery.

c. Successful suicide prevention programs have been demonstrated at the national level as well as at community and school levels.

d. In addition to community level prevention, healthcare settings have a critical role to play in preventing suicide.

e. The language we use surrounding suicide is important, both to correct myths as well as to be respectful of people with lived experience and/or loss.

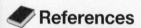

References

1   Stone, D. M., Holland, K. M., Bartholow, B., Crosby, A. E., Davis, S., & Wilkins, N. (2017) *Preventing Suicide: A Technical Package of Policies, Programs, and Practices.* Atlanta, GA: National Center for Injury Prevention and Control, Centers for Disease Control and Prevention.

2   May, P. A., Serna, P., Hurt, L., & Debruyn, L. M. (2005) Outcome evaluation of a public health approach to suicide prevention in an American Indian tribal nation. *Am J Public Health*, 95(7): 1238–44.

3   Wyman, P. A., Brown, C. H., LoMurray, M., et al. (2010) An outcome evaluation of the Sources of Strength suicide prevention program delivered by adolescent peer leaders in high schools. *American Journal of Public Health*, 100(9): 1653–61. doi.org/10.2105/AJPH.2009.190025

4   Wyman, P. A., Pisani, A. R., Brown, C. H., et al. (2020) Effect of the Wingman-Connect Upstream Suicide Prevention Program for Air Force Personnel in Training: A cluster randomized clinical trial. *JAMA network open*, 3(10): e2022532. doi.org/10.1001/jamanetworkopen.2020.22532

5   Knox, K. L., Pflanz, S., Talcott, G. W, et al. (2010) The US Air Force suicide prevention program: Implications for public health policy. *Am J Public Health*, 100(12): 2457–63. doi: 10.2105/AJPH.2009.159871

6   Gouvernement du Québec. (1998) Help for Life: Québec's strategy for preventing suicide. Retrieved from publications.msss.gouv.qc.ca/msss/en/document-000212/.

7   Wilcox, H. C., Kellam, S. G., Brown, C. H., et al. (2008) The impact of two universal randomized first- and second-grade classroom interventions on young adult suicide ideation and attempts. *Drug Alcohol Depend*, 95(Suppl 1): S60-73.

8   Godoy Garraza, L., Kuiper, N., Goldston, D., McKeon, R., & Walrath, C. (2019) Long-term impact of the Garrett Lee Smith Youth Suicide Prevention Program on youth suicide mortality, 2006–2015. *J Child Psychol Psychiatr*, 60: 1142–47. doi: 10.1111/jcpp.13058

9   Lewitzka, U., Sauer, C., Bauer, M., & Felber, W. (2019) Are national suicide prevention programs effective? A comparison of 4 verum and 4 control countries over 30 years. *BMC Psychiatry*, 19: 158. www.ncbi.nlm.nih.gov/pmc/articles/PMC4504869/.

10   Gibbons, R. D., Hur, K., Bhaumik, D. K., & Mann, J. J. (2005) The relationship between antidepressant medication use and rate of suicide. *Arch Gen Psychiatry*, 62(2):165–72.

11   Cavanagh, J. T. O., Carson, A. J., Sharpe, M., & Lawrie, S. M. (2003). Psychological autopsy studies of suicide: A systematic review. *Psychol Med*, 33(3): 395–405.

12   Luoma, J. B., Martin, C. E., & Peason, J. L. (2002). Contact with mental health and primary care providers before suicide: A review of the evidence. *Am J Psychiatry*, 159(6): 909–16.

13   Szanto, K., Kalmar, S., Hendin, H., Rihmer, Z., & Mann, J. J. (2007) A suicide prevention program in a region with a very high suicide rate. *Arch Gen Psychiatry*, 64: 914–20.

14   Ahmedani, B. K., Simon, G. E., Stewart, C., et al. (2014) Health care contacts in the year before suicide death. *J Gen Intern Med*, 29: 870. doi.org/10.1007/s11606-014-2767-3.

15   Frank, R. G., Huskamp, H. A., & Pincus, H. A. (2003) Aligning incentives in the treatment of depression in primary care with evidence-based practice. *Psychiatr Serv*, 54(5): 682–87.

16   Radovic, A., Farris, C., Reynolds, K., Reis, E. C., Miller, E., & Stein, B. D. (2013) Primary care providers' initial treatment decisions and antidepressant prescribing for adolescent depression. *J Dev Behav Pediatr*, 1 doi: 10.1097/DBP.0000000000000008

17   Zuckerbrot, R. A., Cheung, A., Jensen, P. S., Stein, R. E. K., & Laraque, D. (2018) Guidelines for adolescent depression in primary care (GLAD-PC): Part I. practice preparation, identification, assessment, and initial management. *Pediatrics*, 141(3):e20174081.

18   Wintersteen, M. B., & Diamond, G. S. (2013) Youth suicide prevention in primary care: A model program and its impact on psychiatric emergency referrals. *Clin Pract Pediatr Psychol*, 1(3): 295–305. doi: 101037/cpp0000028f

4

Understanding Why: Drivers of Suicide Risk

Ⓐ Introduction

As is the case for all complex health outcomes, there are many risk factors known to increase risk of suicide. In Chapter 6, we will address the clinical assessment of suicide risk, which incorporates risk and protective factors. In the current chapter, we will show how risk factors – health and environmental – weave together and escalate risk at particular moments in a person's life. This chapter will explore how the interaction of biological, psychological, and social/environmental risk factors can increase risk of suicide, differentiating between more enduring and more dynamic factors. We will show how these various factors intersect with life stressors to increase suicide risk. Research related to the global burden of suicide indicates that while cultural factors and available lethal means play a huge role in the suicide risk of a population, many risk and protective factors are shared cross nationally.[1] Understanding, as much as possible, how complex interactions between mental, physical health, and life events pave a path to acute suicide risk, lays the foundation for the preventive measures discussed in the subsequent parts of the book.

Key Point. Understanding how complex interactions between mental health, physical health, and current and past life events pave a path to acute suicide risk, lays the foundation for the preventive measures discussed in the subsequent chapters of the book.

B PRINCIPLES

- A conceptual model for suicide risk is presented, which synthesizes a large body of research about how and when suicide risk increases and how it can be mitigated.

- Risk and protective factors are in somewhat overlapping categories of biological, psychological, and social/environmental. While these are not all as distinct as the categories seem, it is helpful to recognize the kinds of factors that influence risk for suicide.

- Risk and protective factors interact with each other and the interactions are multi-directional.

- Protective factors are critically important and should be identified and encouraged in patient care, however, they are not a guaranteed protection against suicide risk, as protective factors are also dynamic and can be temporarily dismantled during acute crisis. That said, the more robustly the protective factors are in place, generally the more mitigating a role they can play against suicide risk. You can help your patients identify their strongest protective factors to incorporate into their self-management and safety plan.

- Research has illuminated some common features of the perspective of the suicidal mindset. Understanding these findings will help clinicians communicate optimally with patients who are at risk.

- Clinical Takeaways include:
  - o facilitate your patients' insight about their own individual risk and protective factors
  - o continuously filter clinical information, symptoms, and history through the lens of suicide risk assessment so that your assessment remains dynamic and clinical action can be taken appropriately at key times

- Inquiring about suicidal ideation on its own is not an adequate assessment of risk. It is imperative to include risk and protective factors in the clinical suicide risk assessment (outlined in Chapter 6).

Clinical Takeaways

- Facilitate your patients' insights about their own individual risk and protective factors

- Help patients reflect on and hone in on their unique "triggers" for negative spirals or for suicidal ideation

- Continuously filter clinical information, symptoms, and history through the lens of suicide risk assessment so that your suicide risk assessment can be dynamic and clinical action can be taken appropriately at key times

 Model for Understanding Suicide

Psychological Theories. A number of contemporary psychological theories offer frameworks for understanding and explaining why suicide occurs. While a comprehensive overview of theories is beyond the scope of the present volume, a selected review is warranted here. Historically, psychological theories of suicide have focused on suicide as a response to overwhelming pain[2], isolation[3], or hopelessness.[4,5] Most contemporary theories take these factors for granted and shift the focus to explaining why some people who have these experiences move from ideation to action.[6] The Interpersonal Theory of Suicide was the first of these theories and remains the most well-known. The Interpersonal Theory posits that stressors of all kinds lead to suicide when three key phenomena come together and intensify to potentiate behavior: low belongingness (feeling isolated, disconnected, sense of failure to form relationship), burdensomeness (lacking sense of being valuable and valued), and acquired capability (reduced sensitivity to physical pain, fearlessness of death, and ready access to lethal means). The Integrated Motivational-Volitional Model (IMVM) builds upon and recasts the constructs of the Interpersonal Theory.[7] IMVM focuses on entrapment (feeling trapped) and defeat (social humiliation) as primary drivers and explains how people with key background risks and triggering events progress from ideation to behavior. The Three-Step Theory proposes that suicide occurs (i) in the presence of pain and hopelessness, (ii) when the person's pain is greater than their capacity for connection with others, and (iii) they acquire the capability for suicide.[6]

For the purposes of this handbook, we will focus on risk and protective factors that cut across different theories and where the suicide research field provides support. Our goal is to give the reader background knowledge that will be useful both for clinical practice and for delving deeper into any of the psychological theories mentioned above.

● Risk Factors

Psychological autopsy method research studies consistently find multiple risk factors present and interacting just prior to the suicide decedent's untimely death. So, although family members and friends left behind search for reasons for their loved one's death, external observations are not always able to capture the full multi-dimensional changes that were occurring prior to death.

Case Example: John – Part 1

His name was John. He was a 53-year-old executive with a loving wife of more than 20 years, two children in college, a solid career with the same firm, and by his own admission to his doctor, "no reason to be more depressed than any other guy." He had some health issues – he had recently been diagnosed with hypercholesterolemia and borderline diabetes – but they could be addressed. He had been disappointed with being passed over for promotions at work, but he told his wife and friend he had come to terms with his career, saying not everyone can be lucky. A long-time firearm owner having grown up in a hunting and shooting sports-oriented family, he began to feel increasingly ashamed, and like he was a burden on his family. One morning, when his wife was away, he ended his life.

 Risk Factors

What are the drivers of suicide risk? Why do people kill themselves? One narrative that can be dispelled immediately is the idea of the calamitous event, the life tragedy that *on its own* pushes the person over the edge. In fact, suicide is the result of the convergence of several risk factors and life stressors.

Suicide risk factors are characteristics or conditions that increase the chance a person may take their life. Just like someone who is at risk for heart disease because of high blood pressure, or a history of heart disease in the family, some people are at higher risk for suicide than others.

Risk factors can be **more enduring**, i.e., chronic or distal and therefore may seem disconnected to the suicide, such as childhood abuse, or **more dynamic**, i.e., more short term and changing, often proximally connected to the suicide in time and/or space. A dynamic risk factor, for example, could be a recent job stressor or worsening pain condition or depression, both of which have been shown to increase the likelihood of suicide.

Figure 4.1 Model for understanding suicide risk

Multiple risk and protective factors interact dynamically to create periods when risk increases or subsides for an individual. Suicide is not a one-cause/effect phenomenon. While life events can serve as precipitating factors, they are not the sole cause of suicide.

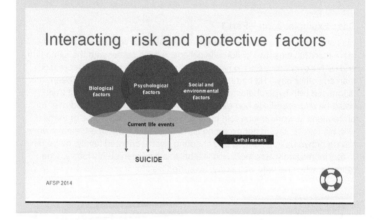

● Biological Risk Factors

The first of the three general categories of risk factors is biological in nature – numerous factors related to the biological make-up of a person, everything from genes to inflammation to brain structure to brain functions such as stress response. Note that the categories are not actually distinct, since many risk and protective factors have several roots and can be quite intertwined. For example, genetics and environmental influences can impact biological (including cellular, neurophysiological, and meta-physiological functions) and psychological traits (including behavioral and cognitive functions).

Biological risk factors tend to be on the more enduring side, especially when chronic in nature. However, even the most seemingly static risk factors can sometimes have the potential to be influenced and mitigated. The most important health/biological risk factors for suicide are **psychiatric conditions**.[1] Those that are known to increase suicide risk, especially when they co-occur with other conditions, include MDD, bipolar disorder, substance use disorders, anxiety disorders, psychotic disorders, borderline personality disorder, impulse control disorders, eating disorders, and PTSD.[8] Research has shown that 85% – 95% of people who die by suicide have a diagnosable mental health condition at the time of their death.[9] Depression is by far the most common mental health condition in general, and is the one that most commonly increases suicide risk, as found in postmortem psychological autopsy studies.[10,11] Bipolar disorder is also associated with a very high risk for suicide, but is less prevalent than depression (3.9% lifetime prevalence for bipolar disorder versus 16.6% for MDD in the general population).[12]

Frequency of Mental Health Conditions in Suicide Decedents[1,9,11]

(Conditions often co-occur in cases of suicide risk therefore the prevalence rates do not add to 100%.)

Major depression (present in 50–60% of suicides)

Bipolar disorder (10%)

Substance use disorders (25%)

Psychosis (15%)

Borderline personality disorder (10%)

Anxiety disorders and PTSD (6%)

Impulse control disorders

Eating disorders

These psychiatric risk factors have been found in suicide studies globally. A study of cross national suicide risk factors showed that, in addition to demographic factors, the presence of a mental disorder, often with psychiatric comorbidity, is one of the most strongly contributing risk factors that remains consistent throughout the world.[13]

A second set of more enduring biological factors relates to genetics, reflected for example in a family history of suicide or mental illness. Researchers have identified several candidate genes that predispose a person to suicide, which could help explain how suicidal behavior is transmitted across generations. This research is in a relatively early phase however, and the results of smaller studies have not been replicated in large-scale genome-wide studies.[14]

There is also epigenetic research indicating that genes and environmental events can interact to increase suicidal behavior. For example, research shows that childhood adversity is associated with the epigenetic regulation of genes, which in turn can alter an individual's stress response system.[15,16] Specifically, an individual's coping and resilience strategies, such as regulating one's emotions or making decisions, can be weakened by early adversity, leading to the potential for increased suicidal behavior in response to stress, even stress that has occurred in the distant past. The literature related to adverse childhood events (ACEs) demonstrates the impact of early stress on multiple outcomes including suicide, mental health, and other health outcomes. The good news is the ACEs studies also demonstrate that risk can be mitigated even in children who have experienced more than six ACEs, for example by the presence of one caring adult in the child's life.[12]

Examples of other more enduring biological risk factors are:

- Neurobiological risk factors (e.g., HPA axis dysfunction, serotonin neurotransmitter systems, other neurotransmitter systems – dopamine, norepinephrine, epinephrine, GABA, glutamate, opioid, and acetylcholine receptors – have also been implicated; stress regulation, fronto-cingulo-striatal network is implicated in suicide risk, reward system, and emotion control, low brain derived neurotrophic factor levels, corticotrophin level alterations, cellular CNS differences in astrocytes and oligodendrocytes)
- Past history of suicidal behavior
- Past history of traumatic brain injury (TBI)

While these risk factors tend to be longer term and less dynamic, they can be mitigated by the epigenetic influence of positive environmental factors like social and family support, and brain health interventions, i.e., effective mental health treatment.

Case Example Continuation: John – Part 2

While John did not show early signs of major depressive disorder, in the two years before his death, he had seemed to family and friends to become more distant, possibly indicating a change in mood that may have stemmed from burgeoning but cloaked clinical depression. Although he dismissed the importance of his loss of promotion, his wife felt that he remained frustrated, possibly interpreting being passed over as a sign of failure or incompetence. Concerning his family history, a key historical biological factor, there had been deaths from both suicide and drug overdose among older relatives. In addition, his mother had shown signs of severe depression after John's brother died in early childhood. His mother's history of depression could represent risk both in terms of genetic history of a mood disorder, as well as related to the psychological, developmental, and environmental impact of being raised by a depressed parent – another known risk factor for poor outcomes such as anxiety and disruptive behavior during childhood and other psychopathology later in life.

4

● More Dynamic Biological Risk Factors

Dynamic risk factors tend to be more short term or proximal, and more readily modifiable. They can serve as an impetus for further destabilization and have the potential to increase suicide risk unless addressed. A recent onset, recurrence, or worsening of a psychiatric condition – for example, a major depressive or bipolar mood episode, or relapse of substance use disorder or a psychotic disorder – could begin a cascade of diminished coping strategies and cognitive changes/distortions, and can "activate" previously "latent" distal risk factors leading to acute suicide risk. A physical medical illness (e.g., pain condition or autoimmune illness flare) could also contribute to increased risk, especially in concert with other suicide risk factors.

New or worsening symptoms related to suicide risk, such as hopelessness, insomnia, agitation, aggression, impulsivity, shame, or burdensomeness, may also serve as proximal biological/psychological risk factors.

Other examples of more dynamic biological risk factors include the following. In each instance the importance of addressing the risk factor as quickly and aggressively as possible cannot be overstated, since the impact on suicide risk is almost never immutable:

- Recently diagnosed or new onset physical health condition (e.g., diabetes, seizure disorder, pain conditions, multiple sclerosis, cancer, infection, HIV/AIDS). These can directly impact physiological brain functioning increasing suicide risk, and can additionally increase suicide risk via the psychological effects of having a newly diagnosed serious health condition.
- Increased use of alcohol or other substances, which have a CNS depressant/ agitating effect, and can worsen other risk factors such as impulsivity and disinhibition.
- New or changing dose of a psychotropic medication – in some cases it can produce usually time-limited side effects of anxiety, agitation, or insomnia. If suicide risk is latent (may not be recognized), negative side effect-related symptoms can increase the potential for suicidal ideation and, rarely, for suicidal behavior. It should be noted, however, that psychiatric medications more often reduce suicide risk when they are used effectively and appropriately monitored. The key is close monitoring at initiation and dose change (see Chapter 9).
- Recent head injury.
- Epigenetic changes (DNA methylation, gene expression) may produce an increased (or decreased) risk for suicide by impacting neurobiology, cognition, or stress regulation. This means that negative experiences such as trauma and

conversely positive experiences such as social support or psychotherapy can actually change gene expression, and can significantly impact an individual's resilience and risk for suicide.

Case Example Continuation: John – Part 3

In the months leading up to his death, John's drinking increased, and his wife noticed that he seemed increasingly "on edge," losing his temper at home more frequently. She thought his sleep had become more fitful. John presented to his primary care physician for weight gain three to four months prior to his death, and he was diagnosed with hypercholesterolemia and borderline diabetes. His increased intake of alcohol and emerging symptoms of insomnia, agitation, and low frustration tolerance may have been the tip of the iceberg heralding underlying mood, cognitive, and coping changes. The newly diagnosed medical conditions may have contributed to his suicide, again via potentially direct biological changes or via individual psychological interpretations of having chronic illness.

Although not illustrated in John's case, one of the strongest predictors of future suicide attempts is a history of suicidal behavior (a prior suicide attempt as a risk factor is considered multifactorial itself, being influenced by several potential layers – biological, psychological, and social/environmental). Research has shown that people who make suicide attempts are significantly (37–40 times) more likely to eventually die by suicide than those who have never attempted suicide before.[11,18] It is also true, however, that the majority of people who survive an attempt do not go on to die by suicide.[19,20] Another predictor of future suicidal behavior is a history of non-suicidal self-injury (NSSI).[21,22] These findings were reported in the 24- and 28-week follow-ups to the Adolescent Depression Antidepressants and Psychotherapy Trial and the Treatment of Selective Serotonin Reuptake Inhibitors-Resistant Depression in Adolescents studies.[21,23,24] So, while NSSI behavior should not be misconstrued as suicidal in intent, and does not necessarily require emergent medical attention, individuals who engage in NSSI can benefit from mental health treatment such as psychotherapy (e.g., Dialectical Behavior Therapy (DBT)) or medications targeting specific diagnoses or symptoms, and sustained treatment can help in short-term ways (symptom and NSSI reduction) as well as long term (can decrease suicide risk.)

● Psychological Risk Factors

Numerous psychological factors can increase suicide risk. It should be emphasized that research shows, as with biological risk factors, that it is not any of these singularly, but rather factors in combination with other risk factors and life events, that increases an individual's risk for suicide.

Psychological risk factors can be **subjectively reported** or **objectively measured**. A good patient history will provide information on previous patterns such as impulsivity, aggression, perfectionism, all-or-none thinking, neuroticism (worrying, overthinking), tendency to become hopeless or anhedonic (the inability to feel pleasure).

Less apparent to the patient but equally important are neurocognitive factors, that are more likely to be revealed through objective measurements. In studies of people with suicidal behavior, compared with controls, they tend to have specific differences in decision making, problem-solving, and other cognitive functions.[25]

These risk factors come into play when they intersect with other risk factors and stressors, such as a current major depressive episode or a traumatic experience or loss.

Specifically, psychological risk factors may operate by:

- Intensifying or distorting negative perceptions and feelings in response to life events and interpersonal interactions
- Increasing the intensity of negative emotions, such as feeling overwhelmed
- Decreasing the ability to flexibly solve problems or seek help
- Increasing the likelihood of responding impulsively rather than pausing to allow intense emotions to recalibrate or to see a future where the problem has subsided
- Deficits in executive functioning, often part of ADHD, mood disorders, and head injuries, produce impairments in the ability to plan multiple steps for complex problems or situations

As a result, some psychological risk factors can be quite invisible or insidious to the individual and possibly to the people in their life. Some are also not necessarily the factors one might expect (e.g., "the least likely person to take their life" – the "high functioning" student or executive, with high degrees of perfectionism and drive, who may also experience recurrent depression or have hidden addiction or PTSD, or "the life of the party, larger than life" individual, which sometimes stems from an underlying bipolar or personality disorder), but they are potentially dangerous when they occur in a patient with other suicide risk factors.

● Distal or Longer Term Psychological Risk Factors

Many distal psychological risk factors, such as neuroticism, perfectionism, or extreme sensitivity to humiliation or rejection, can contribute to a pathway that leads to suicide. Cognitive rigidity, either as a baseline trait or in response to stress, can increase the likelihood that suicide will be narrowed in on and considered the sole solution or way to cope with the current situation.[26]

To summarize, more enduring psychological risk factors include:

- Neuroticism (intrinsic high anxiety trait that is likely inherited, longstanding, usually starting in childhood)
- Perfectionism
- Inflexible or rigid cognitive style
- Innate pessimism/low optimism
- Sensitivity to experiences such as humiliation or perceived rejection leading to bursts of hopelessness or anger

Case Example Continuation: John – Part 4

John did not show any obvious signs of enduring psychological risk factors. However, upon further inspection, he did display a stoic style of coping with disappointment, which while normalized especially for men in many cultures, is not the most adaptive or helpful when mental health needs are on the rise, and especially when other latent suicide risk factors such as family history and childhood adversity are present. While his career setbacks contributed to his suicide, on the surface he did not appear to react to these events, at least overtly or immediately. On the contrary, he may have lacked self-awareness of the psychological impact on his internal dialog and likely tried to tame his despair with alcohol, although this effort likely worsened his mood, sleep, and coping abilities, and buried feelings that resulted in proximal psychological risk states such as shame and hopelessness, as discussed in the next section.

● Proximal or More Dynamic Psychological Risk Factors

Proximal psychological risk factors are often transient, more dynamic psychological experiences that increase risk for suicide. Transition periods in a person's life often trigger psychological shifts, which can exacerbate suicide risk in those with underlying risk. Examples of more dynamic risk factors include:

- Hopelessness
- Burdensomeness

4

- Worthlessness
- Psychological impact of transitions in relationship status, occupation, military, or financial status
- Shame/humiliation related to any current stressor – legal, job, academic
- Sense of failure or loss
- Sense of rejection, disconnection from support network

Case Example Continuation: John – Part 5

Unfortunately, John likely experienced many of these psychological factors in the months and weeks leading to his suicide. After his death, his doctor met with his wife and learned more: that although John mostly did not talk about work at home, that he had brought up his "failure" several times in recent weeks. His wife had dismissed odd, uncharacteristic statements he had made recently about how his father was right after all, that he would never amount to anything (a distal risk factor of parental emotional abuse compounded by a proximal sense of failure and likely diminished self-worth).

These proximal psychological risk factors are especially apparent in John's suicide note in which he stated that he felt he had failed as a husband, had not amounted to what he had thought he was capable of occupationally, and feared that he had become a burden to his family and his employer. He said he believed he actually had no right to complain about his life and so he had tried to keep his feelings of failure and despair to himself.

● Social/Environmental Risk Factors

Social and environmental factors are important in suicide risk and protection and include a range of past or current experiences or exposures. Examples that increase suicide risk include a history of childhood sexual abuse; prolonged psychological stress (e.g., history of trauma, childhood neglect, significant financial/occupational/ relationship stress, or other adverse childhood events or ACEs); cultural beliefs that hinder help seeking or view suicide as an appropriate or acceptable response to specific situations; and critically important – access to lethal means.

● Longer Term Social/Environmental Risk Factors

Distal social/environmental risk factors may be in place but are "latent" in that only in hindsight are we sometimes able to connect the dots. They may be quietly exerting negative impact on health, perceptions, automatic thoughts, and mood/

anxiety over many years, unrecognized but present. They usually do not represent an immediate risk without convergence with the rise in other risk factors like declining mental or physical health, or with a precipitating event occurring. However, once culminating factors or a precipitating event does occur, these longer term social/environmental factors can make a person much more vulnerable to suicide. A common distal social/environmental factor are ACEs, such as physical or sexual abuse, or a childhood marked by neglect or significant early loss. Any prolonged stress, including harassment, bullying, relationship problems, legal problems, and unemployment, can present social/environmental risk as well.

Other specific examples of distal, more enduring social/environmental risk factors include:

- Childhood loss or adversity (e.g., ACEs such as death of parent)
- Prior family discord/violence/rejection
- Growing up with a parent with significant psychiatric illness such as depression, bipolar disorder, or addiction
- Suicide of parent or other family member
- Historical trauma especially for minority/native/indigenous populations
- Cultural or family beliefs that stigmatize mental health and help seeking or view suicide as an acceptable or honorific behavior
- Enduring impoverishment, homelessness

Case Example Continuation: John – Part 6

John grew up with a severely depressed mother and lost a brother when he was young, and although they may seem unrelated, both may have produced psychological and/or epigenetic changes that created risk that contributed to his suicide. Additionally, proximal social/environment risk factors played a role in his death.

● Proximal Social/Environmental Risk Factors

Proximal social/environmental risk factors are recent or current and act as precipitating events or present more near term risk. Layered on a baseline of other underlying distal/enduring risk factors, current exposures or events can serve as suicide precipitants by overwhelming resilience or other healthy coping strategies, or can trigger a quiescent risk factor to become fulminant and suddenly active.

Case Example Continuation: John – Part 7

For example, John may have had genetic risk factors for stress-induced rigid, self-punitive cognitions, which, normally quiescent, became active and forceful, changing his usual way of thinking through and coping with problems, and also leading to a harshly negative self-perception of his life as failure.

Current acute psychosocial stressors, such as legal problems, bullying, unemployment, family conflict, a divorce or a breakup, **and** access to lethal means, can all act as proximal risk factors or "precipitating events."

Proximal social/environment risk factors include:

- The availability of lethal means in one's environment
- Relationship conflict, breakup
- Harassment, bullying
- Loss
- Legal trouble
- Financial crisis
- Exposure to suicide, such as a celebrity suicide or a suicide in the community or among peers, or exposure to graphic or sensationalized accounts of suicide
- Cultural/religious beliefs, which can sometimes reduce the risk, but in some cases can increase it through shaming, rigid, or intolerant beliefs the individual may hear or internalize
- For LGBTQ youth, experiencing rejection by the family or other important community members. Research shows parental accepting behaviors create protection from suicide risk for LGBTQ youth[27]

Case Example Continuation: John – Part 8

John was clearly disappointed with his career, and this disappointment likely snowballed to a complete disenchantment with his life as the alcohol further depressed his brain, and as other distal risk factors likely kicked into action, changing his healthy ways of thinking and coping. He tried to rationalize, both to his wife and his doctor, that he should not be so distressed by the work disappointments, telling his wife that "not everybody can be lucky."

Like many defense mechanisms, stoicism serves an adaptive purpose until it goes too far, keeping the person (and certainly others) from recognizing the distress they are in, and tragically, from being offered support and potentially lifesaving intervention.

One of the most important, potent, and modifiable environmental risk factors is access to a method of killing oneself, which is referred to as access to lethal means. This includes having access to a variety of things, such as firearms, drugs, particular bridges and buildings, a car, coal gas, and pesticides (in Asia), etc.

Every type of lethal means that has been studied has found similar results: When you limit access to lethal means, suicide risk decreases. This is true for methods including coal gas in the UK, pesticides in Asia, medications in the UK, bridge barriers on "suicide hot spot" bridges in multiple countries, and firearms. Therefore, means restriction is considered one of the most effective suicide prevention strategies from a population standpoint.[28,29]

The most common means of suicide death in the USA is firearms; about half of US suicides are by firearms, and the rate is even higher in rural states, for men, and for veterans. As exemplified in the case of John in this chapter, in populations where firearm suicide is common, approaches that make firearms less accessible especially during key times of vulnerability generally lead to lower rates of overall suicide. Substitution of method does not seem to occur in the majority of cases.[30] For example, one study of the Israeli Defense Force found that a policy change requiring service members to leave their firearm on base when they return home for the weekend, led to a 40% decrease in the overall rate of suicide in this cohort.[31] Another way to make firearms less accessible are stronger approaches to secure home storage. A study of firearm suicides among youth, aged 17 and under, occurring over a two-year period in four US states found that 82% used a firearm belonging to a family member, usually a parent.[31] When storage status was noted, about two-thirds of the firearms had been stored unlocked. Among the remaining cases in which the firearms had been locked, the youth knew the combination, where the key was kept, or broke into the cabinet.

Moreover, parents often believe that firearms in the home are adequately "hidden" or that their kids would never use them in a suicide attempt. But studies show parents sometimes underestimate their children's experience handling firearms at home. In a study among firearm-owning parents who reported their children had never handled their firearms at home, 22% of the children, questioned separately, said that they had.[33]

Firearms are not the only way people take their life, so other means must be considered as well. We know that putting time between a person and lethal means reduces suicide risk. For example, installing an inexpensive carbon monoxide sensor that would automatically shut the car off if carbon monoxide reached unsafe levels, would save lives. Installing barriers on bridges deters suicides and in many instances, bridge barriers not only reduced suicides on the bridge, but reduced the suicide rate for the entire region by as much as 40%.[34]

Restricting access to potentially lethal medications reduces suicide risk.[35] It can be as simple as requiring medications with a low therapeutic index to be sold in lesser quantities or blister packaging. Contrary to what may be intuitive, most people who are suicidal, whose chosen method is not accessible, do not find other means and the suicides just never occur; research shows substitution of method does not occur in the majority of cases.[30]

Figure 4.2 Limiting access to lethal means saves lives

Making lethal means for suicide less accessible – at all times for populations and during periods of risk for individuals – reduces suicide risk. This can be accomplished through policy and regulatory changes and making home and work environments as safe as possible (by off-site storage or secure onsite storage of any lethal means).

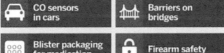

Limiting access to means

CO sensors in cars

Barriers on bridges

Blister packaging for medication

Firearm safety

● **Life Stressors and Precipitating Events**

What science tells us about suicide is that it is not the result of just one cause. Risk factors for suicide can be underlying, latent, perhaps not expressed until a later point in time and often unrecognized as suicide risk mounts. Current life stressors intersect with underlying risk factors to increase suicide risk. Opportunities for potentially lifesaving interventions can be employed if primary care and other health providers recognize these risk factors and their relevance to a patient's suicide risk. This is the main thrust of the suicide risk assessment and care steps, which are covered in practical terms in Chapters 6 and 7.

It is important to emphasize: stressful life events alone do not cause suicide. Instead, current psychosocial stressors can function as precipitating factors when they occur on top of previously mentioned (and usually several) risk factors. These current events can serve as the "final straw" in an increasingly precarious pile-up of converging risk factors, and include a range of stressful events that can be acute or chronic.

Key Point. It important to emphasize: stressful life events alone do not cause suicide. Instead, current psychosocial stressors can function as precipitating factors when they occur on top of previously mentioned (and usually several) risk factors. These current events can serve as the "final straw" in an increasingly precarious pile-up of converging risk factors, and include a range of stressful events that can be acute or chronic.

Acute and Chronic Stressors Play a Role

Acute stressful events include:

- Conflict or breakup of a relationship
- The death of a loved one by any cause
- Loss of a job
- Legal or disciplinary problems
- Financial stress
- Sexual trauma
- Bullying
- Any humiliating or shaming experience

Chronic stress loads known to increase suicide risk include:

- Chronic pain
- Chronic or newly diagnosed physical illness (many chronic medical illness increase suicide risk)
- Traumatic brain injury

- Long-term abusive relationships
- Chronic social rejection
- Family rejection (common experience in LGBTQ youth)
- Unemployment
- Poverty
- Homelessness

Risk Factors for Suicide

We can learn to recognize risk factors as potential clinical targets to reduce risk. Note that no one risk factor on its own is considered the cause of suicide. Rather, multiple risk factors converge and interact to increase risk.

- Psychiatric disorders, especially untreated or undertreated
  - Major depressive disorder (MDD)
  - Bipolar disorder
  - Substance use disorders
  - Psychotic disorders
  - Personality disorder (borderline PD)
  - Eating disorders (anorexia nervosa)
  - PTSD and other anxiety disorders
- Prior suicide attempt
- Hopelessness, mental anguish, or pain (psychological and/or physical)
- Family history of suicide or mental illness
- Early childhood adversity (ACEs such as abuse, neglect, early loss)
- Chronic or severe medical conditions, chronic pain
- Traumatic brain injury (TBI)
- Genetic loading
- Events or losses that cause humiliation, shame, despair, or rejection
- Aggression/impulsivity
- Inflexible, perfectionistic cognitive style
- Exposure to other's suicide or suicidal behavior
- Access to lethal means

Warning Signs

● **Risk Factors versus Warning Signs**

One important distinction is between risk factors and warning signs.

> **Warning signs** are changes in behavior or functioning that signal distress and the potential for **short-term** risk of suicide;
>
> **Risk factors** elevate risk and can be distal/latent/long term (e.g., genetic risk for suicide) or proximal/precipitating events/triggers (e.g., recent bullying or humiliation).

A useful analogous situation is heart disease and death by cardiac arrest due to cardiovascular disease. Risk factors for heart disease include genetic loading/family history, high cholesterol, obesity, tobacco use, unmanaged stress and depression, and lack of physical exercise. However, the presence of these risk factors does not necessarily indicate an immediate risk of a heart attack, whereas warnings signs, such as chest pain, shortness of breath, diaphoresis, and nausea provide signals that myocardial infarction may be imminent.

Clinical Takeaways Related to Warning Signs

Warning signs for escalation in suicide risk include:

- Suicidal ideation – thoughts of or speaking about the possibility of ending their life
- Searching for or acquiring the means to end their life
- Feeling like a burden to others, trapped, or overwhelmed
- Increase in alcohol or substance use
- Anxiety, agitation
- Insomnia
- Hopelessness
- Withdrawing from friends and family
- Dramatic mood changes, irritability, even sudden change to a serene state
- Other uncharacteristic changes in behavior, "personality," or functioning at work, school, or at home
- Giving possessions away

Clinical Takeaways

- Work toward helping your patients gain self-awareness for their own unique triggers, warning signs, and risk factors. (See safety planning in Chapter 7.) The more patients understand "how they tick" and observe their own patterns of both destructive and positive behaviors, relationships, and exposures, the more likely they will be able to incorporate this knowledge into their self-management toolbox.

- For example, you can ask your patient how they believe their spiral downward began. Ask about how their depression might be impacting their work or home life and also if their work or family stress is impacting their depression.

- You can also ask what activities have been the most centering, grounding, or helpful for their mood, anxiety, or suicidal thoughts. Help your patients identify their strongest protective factors and activities to incorporate into their self-management and safety plan.

- Continuously filter clinical information/symptom course, and history through the lens of suicide risk factors so that your risk assessment is ongoing and action can be taken at key times.

 F **Protective Factors**

Protective factors are another important part of an individual's overall picture of risk or mitigation from that risk, and are therefore a key component for suicide risk assessment. There are a host of important protective factors, such as healthy flexible coping, sense of connection, purpose, and feeling supported. Some aspects of resilience are not necessarily even conscious processes.

However, for individuals at high risk in the present moment, even the most solid protective factors can transiently unravel; therefore be wary of putting too much stock in the patient's usual resilience or problem-solving skills, for example, if the patient is in a state of hopelessness and is not coping in his or her usual ways. That said, even extremely at-risk patients often have one or two very powerful reasons for living that help keep them alive, such as a relationship with a child, not wanting to cause the devastating impact of suicide loss for their loved ones, or a particular religious or spiritual belief. It is also important to note that, in the most extreme state of suicidal distress, cognition narrows to a constricted tunnel vision state, which can become fixed on other notions such as a belief that their family would be better off without them. Protective factors should therefore be included as one part of the risk assessment, in the context of recent changes in health, loss/stressors, and changes in patient report and your observed clinical assessment. It can be extremely useful to ask the patient about their reasons for living, and to use the Reasons for Living Inventory developed by Marsha Linehan and colleagues,[36] to ensure protective factors are assessed systematically and can even serve as a therapeutic tool.

That said, protective factors can mitigate a person's risk for suicide, even when several risk factors are present. Even in a state of extreme despair, pain, and hopelessness, most people find a way to reclaim a sense of hope, recover their innate baseline resilience, and find a way to cope in more adaptive ways than taking their life.

Key Point Thinking about Protective Factors in Patient Care

While protective factors are not a guarantee for holding patients steady during periods of high risk, even patients who are at extremely high risk often have one or two very powerful reasons for living that help keep them alive, such as a relationship with a child, not wanting the devastating impact of suicide loss for their loved ones, or a particular religious or spiritual belief.

Therefore, protective factors should be included as one part of the risk assessment. It can be extremely useful to ask the patient about their reasons for living, and to use the Reasons for Living Inventory developed by Marsha Linehan and colleagues,[35] to ensure protective factors are assessed systematically. This approach can also serve as a therapeutic tool.

Most protective factors that mitigate against patients' suicide risk can be grouped into either social/environmental or psychological/cognitive categories.

Social protective factors include:

- Strong support from family and friends
- A sense of connectedness, to people or roles/activities
- Accessing effective mental healthcare
- Cultural or religious beliefs that discourage suicidal behavior, encourage help seeking, or create a strong sense of purpose
- Supportive leaders and peers in professional context

Psychological and cognitive protective factors include positive coping skills that emerge from a wide range of positive cognitive and psychological traits, such as:

- Flexible thinking
- Maintaining hope in the face of difficult circumstances

4

- Optimism
- Finding meaning and purpose even in adversity
- Resilience

Being proactive about mental health, and taking efforts to optimize resilience and other key protective factors specific to the individual, are ways to reduce suicide risk. **One of the strongest protective factors is accessing effective mental healthcare at key high risk times as well as generally throughout their lifetime for mental health conditions and challenges.**

These protective factors can be quite powerful protectors.[37] Unfortunately, when someone is experiencing depression, anxiety, psychosis or substance abuse, protective factors that may normally be strong can erode and weaken usually only temporarily, and often extremely briefly during a crisis period. Having the support of peers, mentors, healthcare providers, friends and family, and retaining the ability to feel that support and connection, can be tremendous protective factors.

Protective factors mitigate against risk for suicide and include:[31]
- Social support
- Sense of connectedness
- Coping skills
- Receiving mental healthcare
- A strong relationship with therapist or other health provider
- Religious or spiritual faith/practice
- Attitudes/beliefs that endorse help seeking as a sign of strength
- Cultural beliefs that do not condone suicide as a reasonable option
- For youth, protective factors include the factors above plus healthy family/ parental dynamic, supportive school and peer environment that promotes growth mindset and healthy coping, messages of acceptance and support, and engaging in mental health treatment as needed

 Dynamic and Interactive: How Convergence of Risk Factors Plays Out

● **An Example of a Set of Risk Factors that Could Converge in a Person who is Suicidal**

One problem with the public perception of suicide is that when someone dies by suicide, it is often the environmental factors that are noted as the cause. These are understandably the factors most visible and easily identified as potential answers to the question of why a person took their life. As shown in Figure 4.3, people see a life event – like a breakup, or bullying, or a job loss – and then they see the person die by suicide, so they might assume the person killed themselves because of that stressful life event.

 Figure 4.3 Understanding Suicide: What others see versus the actual "perfect storm" of converging risk factors

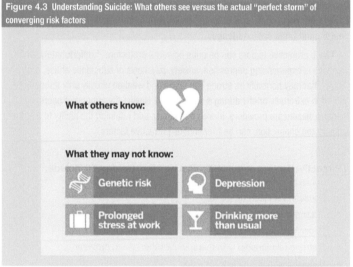

What others know:

What they may not know:

Genetic risk

Depression

Prolonged stress at work

Drinking more than usual

But that's never the full story. What others do not know is that the person who died may have had genetic risks for suicide. Maybe they were suffering from depression and anxiety, and their work life had become increasingly stressful. Their symptoms of depression and anxiety could have made the situation at work even worse, or the work stress could have made their depression worse. Perhaps they had also been drinking more than normal. Cognitive changes during the acute state of distress can lead to distorted perceptions and more rigid problem-solving capacity – all powerful potential contributors to suicide risk. We also know that when a perfect storm of colliding risk factors occurs, particularly when lethal means are accessible, suicide risk escalates. The key is that all of these factors in combination contribute to suicide.

To summarize, a life event can play a precipitating role for suicidal behavior but without other underlying risk factors, life events are not thought to **cause** suicide **on their own**.

H The Perspective of a Suicidal Person

During periods of suicidal thinking, cognition becomes distorted with common feelings of burdening others, oftentimes with increased irritability, depressed mood, and withdrawal. Because they may seem odd or prickly, the natural instinct is to push away or avoid them, when what they really need is a compassionate open-minded person to come alongside and help.

For a suicidal person, thinking becomes limited at the moment of crisis – a state of intense tunnel vision where other options seem unavailable. As a result, a person who is not judging but instead comes across as open and caring can have a powerfully helpful impact on the person in that moment.

Figure 4.4 The perspective of a suicidal person

Research shows that brief moments of suicidal crisis are generally associated with intense physical and/or psychological pain, and a temporary period of cognitive constriction honed in on suicide as an avenue to escape pain.

The Perspective of a Suicidal Person

Crisis point has been reached

Desperate to escape unbearable pain

Thinking becomes irrational

It is important to remember that suicidal feelings are most often temporary. Suicidal feelings can come on intensely and can sometimes pass in minutes or hours. Keeping people safe and making them feel supported can get them through those critical moments and save a life.

There is evidence that putting **time and distance** between an individual who is suicidal and the means to take their lives, can be a lifesaving action. This is why it is so important that we take steps when we know someone is struggling to help keep them safe by working with them to remove lethal means in their environment.

Clinical Takeaways

Clinical Takeaways: Suicidal Ideation, Broader Risk, and Using the Clinical Trajectory

1. **Identify possible risk**. Critical to preventing suicide is the identification of increasing risk. Healthcare providers can facilitate disclosure of suicidal thoughts when patients are struggling, by communicating with compassion and responding with a set of actions (see Chapter 7). Realize that even high functioning patients who have been in good health can become at risk. Suicide risk does not have a cookie cutter prototype of patient.

2. **Develop a more sensitive radar for patients who are struggling silently. Many patients present without spontaneous declaration of their suicidal thoughts but rather with subtle cues that may only allude to their despair**. It is critically important to follow patients' clues hinting at hopelessness or thoughts of ending their life to uncover suicide risk. For a variety of reasons including stigma and shame, and not knowing if/when/with whom it is "safe" to disclose suicidal thoughts, some patients will not disclose their suicidal thoughts, spontaneously or even when asked. As a result, other methods should be used to detect a patient with deteriorating mental health who is becoming at risk of suicide. A further complication is that due to the dynamic nature of suicide risk, a person may not have suicidal thoughts in one moment, but may become suicidal at a later moment; in this case, there may be risk factors that may cue a referral or closer follow-up, even though suicidal ideation is not present at the time of the office visit.

3. **Suicidal ideation indicates risk but on its own is not sufficient to assess risk**. It is important to realize that suicidal thoughts are common (some studies find lifetime occurrence as high as 60% and one-week point prevalence up to 17% in the general population),[1,2] therefore on its own **suicidal ideation does not indicate high suicide risk. It does however signal the need to assess suicide risk in a more thorough manner. Suicidal ideation is neither sensitive nor specific enough to be the only factor in determining a patient's current risk**. While a sensitive indicator of distress is critically important to detect and respond to, suicidal thinking is so commonplace in the population that the decision whether to hospitalize for example, should not be made solely on the presence of suicidal thoughts. Other risk factors must be considered part

of risk assessment in order to identify level of acuity. This risk assessment process is outlined in detail in Chapter 6.

4. **Gain a sense of the patient's trajectory including protective factors.** Are symptoms and stressors worsening over several days or weeks, and are there one or two particular symptoms that seem to be the most potent in terms of creating distress or hopelessness for the patient? Are their protective factors and reasons for living still strongly intact? Are foreseeable changes coming that will help broaden your understanding of their risk or supports in place? Engaging the patient in an open dialog about their perspective can uncover key information that may tip the assessment/plan in either direction.

5. **Consider other historical factors** such as prior attempts, hospitalizations, previous episodes of suicidal ideation, family history of suicide or attempts, and history of abuse, can all be relevant. Additionally, psychosocial factors related to the patient's job, marriage, pending legal issues, and finances can all be part of a clinical presentation; discussions about these issues can help elicit and possibly help engage the patient and others in a plan to alleviate the patient's sense of hopelessness.

KEY TAKEAWAYS

a. A model for understanding how suicide risk increases and also how it can be mitigated is important to understand and integrate into clinical thinking and care.

b. Risk and protective factors are dynamic and interact with one another.

c. Protective factors are critically important, however, they are not a guaranteed protection against suicide risk, as protective factors are also dynamic and can be temporarily dismantled during acute crisis. That said, the more robust protective factors are in place, generally the more mitigating they can be against suicide risk.

d. The perspective of the suicidal mind must be considered in order to communicate effectively with someone at-risk.

e. Clinical takeaways, including continuously filtering new and historical clinical information and symptoms through the lens of suicide risk assessment, are important so that action can be taken appropriately.

f. Suicidal ideation on its own is not an adequate assessment of risk. It is imperative to include risk, protective factors, and foreseeable changes into the clinical suicide risk assessment and care plan.

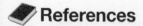 # References

1   Bertolote, J. M., & Fleischmann, A. (2002) Suicide and psychiatric diagnosis: a worldwide perspective. *World Psychiatry: Official Journal of the World Psychiatric Association (WPA)*, 1(3): 181–85.

2   Shneidman, E. S. (1993) *Suicide as Psychache: A Clinical Approach to Self-Destructive Behavior*. Northfield, NJ: Jason Aronson.

3   Durkheim, E. (1951) *Suicide: A Study in Sociology*. New York, NY: Free Press. (Original work published 1897).

4   Abramson, L. M., Alloy, L. B., Hogan, M. E., et al. (2000) The hopelessness theory of suicidality. In T. Joiner & M. D. Rudd (Eds.), *Suicide Science: Expanding the Boundaries* Norwell, MA: Kluwer Academic Publishers, 17–32.

5   Beck, A. T. (1967) *Depression: Clinical, Experimental, and Theoretical Aspects*. New York, NY: Harper & Row.

6   Klonsky, E. D., & May, A. M. (2015) The three-step theory (3ST): A new theory of suicide rooted in the "ideation-to-action" framework. *International Journal of Cognitive Therapy*, 8(2): 114–29.

7   O'Connor, R. C. (2011) Towards an integrated motivational-volitional model of suicidal behaviour. International handbook of suicide prevention: *Research, Policy and Practice*, 1: 181–98.

8   Hawton, K., Hall, S., Simkin, S., et al. (2003) Deliberate self-harm in adolescents: a study of characteristics and trends in Oxford, 1990–2000. *J Child Psychol Psychiatry*, 44(8): 1191–98.

9   Cavanaugh, J. T., Carson, A. J., Sharpe, M., & Lawrie, S. M. (2003) Psychological autopsy studies of suicide: a systematic review. *Psychol Med*, 33(3): 395–405.

10 Nordentoft, M., Mortensen, P. B., & Pedersen, C. B. (2011) Absolute risk of suicide after first hospital contact in mental disorder. *Arch Gen Psychiatry*, 68(10): 1058–64. doi: 10.1001/archgenpsychiatry.2011.113

11 Harris, E. C., & Barraclough, B. (1997) Suicide as an outcome for mental disorders. A meta-analysis. *Br J Psychiatry*, 170: 205–28.

12 Kessler, R. C., Mickelson, K. D., & Williams, D. R. (1999) The prevalence, distribution, and mental health correlates of perceived discrimination in the United States. *J Health Soc Behav*, 40(3): 208–30.

13 Nock, M. K., Borges, G., Bromet, E. J., et al. (2008) Cross-national prevalence and risk factors for suicidal ideation, plans and attempts. *Br J Psychiatry*, (2): 98–105. doi: 10.1192/bjp.bp.107.040113

14 Perlis, R. H., Huang, J., Purcell, S., et al. (2010) Genome-wide association study of suicide attempts in mood disorder patients. *Am J Psychiatry*, 167(12): 1499–507.

15 McGowan, P. O., Sasaki, A., D'Alessio, A. C., et al. (2009) Epigenetic regulation of the glucocorticoid receptor in human brain associates with childhood abuse. *Nature Neuroscience*, 12(3): 342–48.

16 Turecki, G., Ernst, C., Jollant, F., Labonté, B., & Mechawar, N. (2012) The neurodevelopmental origins of suicidal behavior. *Trends Neurosci*, 35 (1):14–23. doi: 10.1016/j.tins.2011.11.008. Epub 2011 Dec 15.

17 Felitti, V. J., Anda, R. F., Nordenberg, D., et al. (1998) Relationship of childhood abuse and household dysfunction to many of the leading causes of death in adults: The Adverse Childhood Experiences (ACE) Study. *Am J Prev Med*, 14(4): 245–58. doi: 10.1016/S0749-3797(98)00017-8

18   Olfson, M., Wall, M., Wang, S., Crystal, S., Gerhard, T., & Blanco, C. (2017) Suicide following deliberate self-harm. *Am J Psychiatry*, 174(8): 765–74. doi: 10.1176/appi.ajp.2017.16111288

19   Hawton, K., Zahl, D., & Weatherall, R. (2003) Suicide following deliberate self-harm: long-term follow-up of patients who presented to a general hospital. *Br J Psychiatry*, 182(6): 537–42.

20   Fedyszyn, I. E., Erlangsen, A., Hjorthøj, C., Madsen, T., & Nordentoft, M. (2016) Repeated suicide attempts and suicide among individuals with a first emergency department contact for attempted suicide: a prospective, nationwide, Danish register-based study. *J Clin Psychiatry*, 77(6): 832–40. doi: 10.4088/JCP.15m09793

21   Asarnow, J. R., Porta, G., Spirito, A., et al. (2011). Suicide attempts and nonsuicidal self-injury in the treatment of resistant depression in adolescents: findings from the TORDIA study. *Journal of the American Academy of Child and Adolescent Psychiatry*, 50(8): 772–81.

22   Prinstein, M. J., Nock, M. K., Simon, V., Aikins, J. W., Cheah, C. S., & Spirito, A. (2008) Longitudinal trajectories and predictors of adolescent suicidal ideation and attempts following inpatient hospitalization. *Journal Consult Clin Psychol*, 76(1): 92–103.

23   Emslie, G. J., Mayes, T., Porta, G., et al. (2010) Treatment of Resistant Depression in Adolescents (TORDIA): week 24 outcomes. *Am J Psychiatry*, 167(7): 782–91.

24   Brent, D. A., Emslie, G. J., Clarke, G. N., et al. (2009) Predictors of spontaneous and systematically assessed suicidal adverse events in the treatment of SSRI-resistant depression in adolescents (TORDIA) study. *Am J Psychiatry*, 166(4): 418–26.

25   Williams, G. E., Daros, A. R., Graves, B., et al. (2015) Executive functions and social cognition in highly lethal self-injuring patients with borderline personality disorder. *Personality Disorders: Theory, Research, and Treatment*, 6(2): 107–16. doi: 10.1037/per0000105

26   Jager-Hyman, S., Cunningham, A., Wenzel, A., Mattei, S., Brown, G. K., & Beck, A. T. (2014) Cognitive distortions and suicide attempts. *Cognitive Therapy and Research*, 38(4): 369–74. doi. org/10.1007/s10608-014-9613-0

27   Ryan, C., Russell, S. T., Huebner, D., Diaz, R., & Sanchez, J. (2010) Family acceptance in adolescence and the health of LGBT young adults. *External J Child Adolesc Psychiatr Nurs* 23(4): 205–13.

28   Gunnell, D., & Miller, M. (2010). Strategies to prevent suicide. *BMJ*, 341:157–8.

29   Mann J.J., Michel C.A., Auerbach R.P. (2021) Improving suicide prevention through evidence-based strategies: A systematic review. *Am J Psychiatry*, doi:10.1176/appi.ajp.2020.20060864

30   Barber, C. W., & Miller, M. J. (2014) Reducing a suicidal person's access to lethal means of suicide. *Am J Prev Med*, 47(3S2): S264–72.

31   Lubin, G., Werbeloff, N., Halperin, D., Shmushkevitch, M., Weiser, M., & Knobler, H. Y. (2010) Decrease in suicide rates after a change of policy reducing access to firearms in adolescents: a naturalistic epidemiological study. *Suicide Life Threat Behav*, 40: 421–4. doi: 10.1521/ suli.2010.40.5.421

32   Johnson, R. M., Barber, C., Azrael, D., Clark, D. E., & Hemenway, D. (2010) Who are the owners of firearms used in adolescent suicides? *Suicide Life Threat Behav*, 40(6): 609–11.

33   Baxley, F., & Miller, M. (2006) Parental misperceptions about children and firearms. *Arch Pediatr and Adolesc Med*, 160(5): 542–47.

34   Bennewith, O., Nowers, M., & Gunnell, D. (2007) Effect of barriers on the Clifton suspension bridge, England, on local patterns of suicide: Implications for prevention. *Br J Psychiatry*, 190: 266–67.

35 Gunnell, D., Hawton, K., Bennewith, O., et al. (2013) A multicentre program of clinical and public health research in support of the *National Suicide Prevention Strategy for England*. Southampton (UK): NIHR Journals Library.

36 Linehan, M. M., Goodstein, J. L., Nielsen, S. L., & Chiles, J. A. (1983) Reasons for staying alive when you are thinking of killing yourself: the reasons for living inventory. *J Consult Clin Psychol*, 51: 276–86.

37 Malone, K. M., Oquendo, M. A., Haas, G. L., Ellis, S. P., Li, S., & Mann, J. J. (2000) Protective factors against suicidal acts in major depression: Reasons for living. *Am J Psychiatry*, 157(7): 1084–88.

SECTION 2
Clinical Risk Assessment and Care

5

Collaborative Connections

A Introduction: The Challenge and Opportunity

Suicide concerns can present themselves in a wide range of
healthcare situations, from routine screening to dealing with a
person in the aftermath of a suicide attempt, and can even arise
spontaneously when talking with a person struggling with suicidal
thoughts.

When engaging with persons at risk for suicide, healthcare professionals have an
opportunity to make a real difference in the life of the patient. However, the situation
can place a great deal of pressure on those trying to help. When dealing with a person
struggling with suicidal thoughts, a variety of concerns might arise:

- The clinician cares about the person and worries about their safety.
- They now feel personally responsible for the safety of the person.
- There are time-consuming steps to take and documentation to fill out.
- The clinician may be worried about being blamed or held legally liable if
  something goes wrong.

Settings: Acute Services

Acute services teams have a unique opportunity to support and care for individuals with mental illness who are often at a very vulnerable point in their lives. But time demands, patient volume, and the sheer number of different risks and problems that teams are responsible for addressing can make it hard to take the time for caring interactions that will promote honest disclosure.

These pressures can make it hard to remain focused and to maintain the kind of concerned but calm presence that will help patients through this difficult situation.

This chapter focuses on the core goal of **Connecting**. Forming a meaningful connection with the patient serves as the foundation for all other steps that need to be taken in a medical setting to support a person with suicide concerns.

B PRINCIPLES

- Forming a genuine connection with an at-risk person not only helps with understanding but is also a preventive measure in and of itself. Maintaining a concerned and calm presence is essential to achieving this goal.

- Ask directly about suicide using a standard approach and with the goal of understanding the person's experience and the purpose that suicidal thinking serves for them.

- Involve family and other support people early and often.

- Connecting with family members can cast light on the at-risk person's experiences and can also show how family members can support them.

- Approach conversations as a route toward finding common goals with the shared aim of working together to help the person feel better.

- Recognize that while medical professionals see suicide as a problem, people with suicidal thoughts see it as a potential last resort solution to problems.

- Validate the desire to be free from pain and offer hope that the person can get better.

- Express a personal and institutional commitment not just to the person's safety but to their full recovery.

- Finish conversations with a strong emphasis on hope.

Rationale

Forming a meaningful connection is a vital part of suicide prevention. A lack of connection to others was one of the first common problems identified by early observers of suicide,[1] and contemporary studies have repeatedly confirmed the link between suicide risk and a person feeling disconnected from those around them.[2–5]

The practical task of promoting a feeling of connection with professional helpers and with those in the person's natural support network is a critical component of almost every effective psychosocial intervention.

This chapter will explain key aspects of how to form a connection using three keywords that can serve as a reminder of core skills and practices:

Ask, Collaborate, and Commit.

 Ask

Ask refers to:

1. **Asking** directly about suicide with a standard approach

and

2. **Asking** with the goal of understanding the person's experience

Significant progress has been made in recent years toward the use of standardized tools and measures for assessing suicidal thoughts and behavior (see Chapter 6 for a review of these measures). However, sticking rigidly to the wording used in a validated measure does not guarantee an open and honest response, and can sometimes even be counterproductive. The goal of an assessment is to understand what the person is thinking and feeling. While asking valid questions on a scale is important,[6] it is equally important to remember that the person with suicide concerns is an individual with unique experiences. Excessive focus on a standardized tool can sometimes obscure the personalized suffering that underlies and prompts yes/no responses.

In order to provide effective care to a person at risk of suicide, it is vital to form a connection on a human level. The best way to form such a connection is to **ask** questions that will help provide a personal understanding of how the individual feels.[7]

Example Questions

- *"Are you having thoughts about suicide?"*
- *"Where are you when you're having these thoughts?"*
- *"What's it like?"*

How these questions are asked can have a significant impact on the connection that is formed with the person. In asking questions, it is important to honor the person's experience of suicidal thoughts and behavior. The goal is to find out ***what it is like for them and what purpose the suicidal thinking serves for this particular individual***.

If somebody says that they have had a specific thought about suicide or have a plan for ending their life, one line of questioning is to ask them what it is like to experience having such thoughts.

- *"Does that make you feel worried?"*
- *"Does that ever scare you?"*
- *"Have you been keeping that inside?"*
- *"How does that comfort you?"*

Connecting with family members is also important. Engagement with the thoughts and experiences of family members can help the medical professional understand what they are going through. This will make it easier to communicate with them and to work together to take planning actions. Asking about the person's experiences is the first step toward forming this connection.

- *"What was it like for you to hear that?"*
- *"Does that feel overwhelming?"*
- *"Does that scare you?"*

Settings: Acute Care

Those who work in inpatient and other acute settings choose to work with people who have the most serious mental health needs, often at their most painful moments. Asking about the person's suffering fits well with this core mission and its related skills.

Although these ways of asking may be unfamiliar, the concern behind them is consistent with what motivates much of our work as healthcare professionals: a direct concern for what the patient is experiencing. When dealing with suicide risk, it can help to refocus on the human dimension of medicine and to center approaches on the fundamental interaction of empathizing with the person who is being cared for.

Family and Support People Are Central not Collateral

We often describe family members and other support as "collateral contacts." But think about your own relationships with family and friends. Are these people collateral to you?

5

E Collaborate

Collaborate refers to:

1. Finding shared goals and common ground with the suicidal person

and

2. Involving family and other support people early and often

Lived Experience Perspective

"When I think about what I really wanted when I was in a suicidal mindset, it was very simple: I wanted to end the pain I was in. When you're feeling that hopeless, you can't see any other way out of the pain, and you aren't able to put into words, 'I just want to feel better.'"

When talking with someone about their suicidal thoughts or plans, there is a potential disconnect between the healthcare professional's perspective of suicide as a **problem**, and the person's preoccupation with suicide as a potential **solution**. In this context, the healthcare professional's natural focus is on "keeping you safe." By contrast, the priority of the person at risk is the series of difficulties, trauma, and stress that have pushed them to a point at which they feel that ending their lives would be better than continuing to live. For them, suicide seems to be a way of escaping from pain and suffering.[8]

While these two views of suicide might seem to be at odds with one another, both parties in fact want exactly the same thing: for the suicidal person to **feel better**.

To resolve this apparent tension and remove a potential obstacle to forming a meaningful connection, the caregiver needs to:

1. Strongly validate the desire to be free of pain and
2. Offer real hope that the person can get better

This approach is consistent with one of the most heavily researched suicide-specific therapies,[9] Dialectical Behavior Therapy (DBT). In DBT, the fundamental therapeutic concept is the balancing of radical acceptance with a push for radical change.[10,11] We have the opportunity to practice this philosophy in everyday interactions with the person who is suffering. Accept and validate their pain – avoiding the temptation to "talk them out of it" – and hold onto the hope that the person themselves cannot yet see.

F │ Commit

The final aspect of connecting is the skill of **committing** to the person's full recovery. This involves expressing a personal commitment to this goal as well as expressing the commitment of the team or organization to which the clinician belongs.[12,13]

Persons at risk often hear caregivers talk about a commitment to their safety. However, it is less common to hear a commitment to moving forward with them beyond immediate safety concerns and toward living a life that is rich and abundant once again. Healthcare workers may feel this commitment on the inside, but it is important for these feelings to be vocalized.

"This isn't going to be easy, and it might take trying a few different things before we find the right combination of help, support, and steps you can take, but if you stick with it we will stick with you all the way."

Challenge and Opportunity

In some cases, you may only meet a person struggling with suicidal thoughts once. What is the best way to support them in such circumstances? It is critical for all members of a team, an organization, or even an entire healthcare region to be on the same page with a common framework so that when you tell a person something you can have confidence that the whole system will back you up.

"I might only be here with you today, but I'm one person in a whole system of people who are also committed not just to your safety but to achieving the best possible outcome for you."

Settings: Acute Services

Keeping patients safe is an important part of the mission. But while safety is necessary, the job of an inpatient hospital is to start patients on their path to recovery.

Challenges to Connecting

5

While these skills are all used in other contexts in the healthcare workplace, they can often seem harder to apply in the context of suicide risk. When dealing with the potential for the death of a patient, feelings of personal responsibility can become overwhelming and this sense can compound with personal experiences, time pressures, and fear of liability to create obstacles to forming a connection.[14,15]

We are affected by:

- Personal experiences
- Liability issues and concerns (legal and personal/moral)
- Feelings of helplessness
- Time pressures (documentation, etc.)
- Ethnic and family cultural differences
- Patients who are hard to relate to

Caregivers have a number of options when faced with such obstacles to forming a connection:

Consult. Consultation with colleagues often provides new insights into problems and ways of resolving them. Consultation is also one of the most powerful medicolegal protections available and, as such, can help relieve pressures relating to liability. Cultural consultation can also help in navigating unfamiliar cultural or social frameworks. Indeed, consultation is such a valuable tool that one evidence-based suicide treatment[11] requires team members to have regular consultations about their own feelings with a specialized consultation team.

Consider therapy. When encouraging people to seek help, caregivers may also benefit from therapeutic approaches themselves, particularly if the pressure of dealing with suicide becomes hard to manage or if they have had personal experiences relating to suicide.

Lean on the framework. It is important to remember that there is a treatment framework available to use – healthcare professionals do not have to develop a new approach each time they deal with a person who is at risk of suicide. Following the framework is both more efficient and ensures that caregivers are legally protected.

Identify missed connections. If a caregiver feels that they are not connecting with the person they are trying to help, it is never too late to try again. The ability to identify and recognize a connection issue also makes it possible to try to reconnect.

Ask. When it is difficult to understand a cultural or personal dimension in someone's experience, or when that person seems hard to relate to as an individual, it can be useful to return to the first concept discussed in this chapter and **ask** the person to say more about their situation and what they are experiencing.

● Malignant Alienation

Forming connections is especially important for patients who can be hard to like. The term malignant alienation has been used to describe patients, especially in group settings, who are disliked and rejected both by other patients and by staff. At least one study of completed inpatient suicide showed that these people were more likely to kill themselves. One remedy for malignant alienation is to gather the clinical team together to review the person's family tree. This procedure often reveals a great deal of trauma and adversity in the person's background and uncovering this information can generate a greater understanding of the individual and of their challenging behaviors. This provides an opportunity to create a different therapeutic experience for somebody who may have gone through their whole life being kept at arms-length by other people.[16]

Early Career Professionals Need Stories of Hope

Short training rotations often do not allow students to follow people from moments of crisis through to recovery. The emphasis in clinical rounds and other treatment team meetings trainees attend tends to be on immediate safety or on those who are not getting better. We need to remind students that, while of course we want people we work with to be safe, we have much more to offer as well. As a teacher, you can point to solid research on the effectiveness of treatments. As a student or someone early in their career who has not yet been fortunate enough to see someone recover, you can ask your supervisors and teachers for their stories. In either case, it is important not to allow the necessary constraints of training programs to undermine confidence in the ability of healthcare professionals to make a difference.

Communicating Hope

Finishing with a strong emphasis on hope is important. If there is one thing the person should take away from their initial interaction, it is that they **can** get better.

The skills used in responding to suicide risk build on the same skills medical professionals use every day in treating their other patients: Asking about experiences, collaborating toward the common goal of feeling better, and offering confidence. Once the fears and concerns that emerge when dealing with suicide are overcome, it is simply a matter of applying familiar skills in this challenging and rewarding area.

 Patient Perspective

"When I was in the hospital, I can't tell you how many times people told me that their goal was to keep me safe. While I appreciated the emphasis on safety, for me it missed the point. I had lost my career and I was convinced my life was over. I didn't want to be safe, I wanted to escape. One time, however, I heard something different. A nurse, on his way out of my room, leaned over and said, "You can beat this." That made a difference. Hearing from one nurse that I could beat this meant a lot."

 KEY TAKEAWAYS

In order to Connect: **Ask**, **Collaborate**, and **Commit**.

 Figure 5.1 Ask, Collaborate, and Commit

Ask
... directly, using standardized items
... about the person's experience

Collaborate
... around the common goal of feeling better
... early and often with family, friends, and others

Commit
... to full recovery

Bringing these together makes it clear to the person thinking about suicide that:

- You are seeking to **understand** the desire behind suicidal thinking and behavior
- You share the **common goal** of reducing suffering
- You are **committed** to that goal, and, with cooperation and openness from the person and their family, you believe that they have what is needed to achieve that goal

I Understand

*"I can understand that, with all you've been through, it makes sense that you'd want to search for some way, any way, to be free of that pain.
I share that same goal."*

and

There is Hope

"Based on my own experience, as well as decades of research, I can tell you this: if you can come in good faith and work with this team and the plans we identify together, then you can feel better."

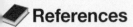

References

1   Durkheim, E. (1951) *Suicide: A Study in Sociology*. Trans. J. A. Spaulding and G. Simpson, New York: The Free.

2   Dervic, K., Brent, D. A., & Oquendo, M. A. (2008) Completed suicide in childhood. *Psychiatric Clinics*, 31(2): 271–91.

3   Joiner, T. E. Jr, & Van Orden, K. A. (2008) The interpersonal–psychological theory of suicidal behavior indicates specific and crucial psychotherapeutic targets. *International Journal of Cognitive Therapy*, 1(1): 80–89.

4   Trout, D. L. (1980) The role of social isolation in suicide. *Suicide Life-Threat Behav*, 10(1): 10–23.

5   Van Orden, K. A., Witte, T. K., & Cukrowicz, K. C. (2010) The interpersonal theory of suicide. *Psychol Rev*, 117(2): 575–600.

6   Kendall, P. C., & Frank, H. E. (2018) Implementing evidence-based treatment protocols: Flexibility within fidelity. *Clinical Psychology: Science and Practice*, 25(4): e12271.

7   Pompili, M. (2010) Exploring the phenomenology of suicide. *Suicide Life-Threat Behav*, 40(3): 234–44.

8   Shneidman, E. S. (1993) *Suicide as Psychache: A Clinical Approach to Self-Destructive Behavior*. Lanham, MD: Jason Aronson.

9   Panos, P. T., Jackson, J. W., Hasan, O., & Panos, A. (2014) Meta-analysis and systematic review assessing the efficacy of dialectical behavior therapy (DBT). *Research on Social Work Practice*, 24(2): 213–23.

10 Linehan, M. M. (1993) *Cognitive-Behavioral Treatment of Borderline Personality Disorder*. New York: Guilford Press.

11 Robins, C. J., Schmidt, H. III, & Linehan, M. M. (2004) Dialectical behavior therapy: synthesizing radical acceptance with skillful means. In S. C. Hayes, V. M. Follette, & M. M. Linehan (Eds.), *Mindfulness and Acceptance: Expanding the Cognitive-Behavioral Tradition*. New York: Guilford Press, 30–44.

12 Leamy, M., Bird, V., Le Boutillier, C., Williams, J., & Slade, M. (2011) Conceptual framework for personal recovery in mental health: systematic review and narrative synthesis. *Br J Psychiatry*, 199(6): 445–52.

13 Connell, J., Brazier, J., O'Cathain, A., Lloyd-Jones, M., & Paisley, S. (2012) Quality of life of people with mental health problems: a synthesis of qualitative research. *Health and Quality of Life Outcomes*, 10(1): 138.

14 Sprang, G., Clark, J. J., & Whitt-Woosley, A. (2007) Compassion fatigue, compassion satisfaction, and burnout: Factors impacting a professional's quality of life. *Journal of Loss and Trauma*, 12(3): 259–80.

15 McAdams, C. R. III, & Foster, V. A. (2000) Client suicide: Its frequency and impact on counselors. *Journal of Mental Health Counseling*, 22 (2): 107–21.

16 Watts, D., & Morgan, G. (1994) Malignant alienation. Dangers for patients who are hard to like. *Br J Psychiatry*, 164(1): 11–15.

6

Prevention-Oriented Suicide Risk Assessment

Ⓐ Introduction

Information about specific risk and protective factors for assessments is presented in Chapter 4. In this chapter, we present selected clinical considerations for integrating and synthesizing information gathered about well-known risk factors so that it can be used to improve our understanding of the individual person and to drive plans and responses.

What Is Your Role?

Depending upon your role, you may have responsibility for different parts of an assessment process. Can you identify your role? Are you gathering information and passing it on to others? Are you responsible for synthesizing and acting on risk assessment? Even if you are only responsible for a small part of the overall process, it will be useful to understand the whole framework so that you can contribute effectively to a team.

The first part of this chapter will provide a repeatable structure for gathering and communicating key information about the person's life and experiences that provide a context for understanding suicidal thoughts and behavior.

6

The second part focuses on detection and assessment of suicidal ideation, behavior, and risk. This includes structured screening and assessment, interviewing techniques, and emerging methods that do not rely on self-report.

The third part of this chapter covers prevention-oriented risk formulation – a framework for synthesizing and communicating about risk in a way that is anchored and actionable in a particular setting and in a particular individual's life.

Figure 6.1 Prevention-oriented risk formulation

The left side of the figure provides a repeatable structure for gathering and communicating data that informs assessment. The right side of the figure provides a framework for synthesizing and communicating about risk in a way that is anchored and actionable in a particular setting and in a particular individual's life.

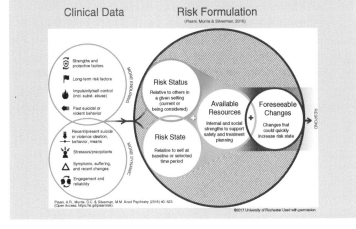

B PRINCIPLES

- Assessment of suicide risk must go beyond just questions about suicidal thoughts and plans. The goal of an assessment is to **understand** suicide risk in the context of the whole person and their situation.

- Routine use of structured screening tools helps ensure consistent assessment and decreases the chances that key questions will be missed.

- Protocols and techniques for responding to a positive screen are just as important as the instrument you choose.

- Structured screening alone will miss many people at risk, often including those with the highest intent. The validity techniques covered in this chapter enhance the accuracy of answers to screening questions.

- When assessing data for a risk assessment, it is important to consider the level of engagement of the person and the reliability of their answers.

- Prevention-oriented risk formulation helps healthcare professionals develop a personalized and context-specific understanding of the dynamics of a person's situation, and helps communicate this complex and changing situation to others.

- Risk formulations start from understanding the enduring and dynamic factors underlying suicide risk: strengths and protective factors; long-term risk factors; impulsivity and self-control; stressors and precipitants; symptoms, suffering, and recent changes.

- The purpose is not prediction, but planning. The goal of risk formulation is to promote communication, collaboration, and action among professionals, patients, and families in order to reduce risk.

- While stratification into high, medium, or low risk can be useful, more nuanced formulations will consider the person's risk relative to broader populations (risk status) and their risk relative to themselves at other times (risk state).

- More important than the level of risk is identifying what could exacerbate risk and what resources are available to help in crisis and treatment.

Understanding the Context for Suicide Risk

The first part of this chapter will introduce a structure for understanding and communicating contextual information about suicide risk. Having a structure for person-specific information helps organize the elements of a person's story so that it can be used to drive responses and provide a common "language" for communicating with colleagues inside and outside one's organization, in team meetings and hand-offs, and in health record documentation.

● Enduring versus Dynamic Factors

Information relevant to suicide risk can be organized loosely into factors that are more enduring and factors that are more dynamic. When first working with someone, it is critical to understand their history and background. Enduring factors emerge from listening to a person's history. Over time, tracking changes in dynamic factors is critical for identifying specific periods of vulnerability.

● Enduring Factors

Strengths and Protective Factors

Chapter 4 listed some statistically important protective factors. In addition to these, it is helpful to identify things that make a person feel unique or good about themselves, whether or not these are documented epidemiological protective factors. Does the person have talents or hobbies? Do their friends say they have a great sense of humor? Do they have a strong family support system or a connection to a religious community?

Patient Perspective

*"Sometimes you'll encounter a person who can't seem to say anything positive about themselves. That was me when I was thinking about suicide. I thought the world would be better off without me, and I didn't see anything good about myself. If you are working with someone like that, you could ask what positive things **other people** might say about them."*

Gathering information about what is strong, special, and unique about a person and about what is important to them helps all involved to see the at-risk person as more than just a diagnosis or a list of problems. Eliciting strengths helps forge a connection between clinician and patient and provides insights into how the patient sees themselves or their contribution to the world. Understanding how a person sees their core strengths provides insights into what future changes or losses might lead to increased risk and provides a starting place for protective plans.

Case Example: Starting with Strength in Case Presentations

Jessica is a 14-year-old girl.

Traditional case presentations start with the problem: "This is a 14-year-old girl with a long history of depression, multiple foster-care placements, presents with agitation."

But with only a little extra effort, we can set the scene with strengths: "Jessica is a 14-year-old girl who loves to sing and draws cartoons that all the other kids love."

Beginning with the person's strengths and uniqueness evokes a different picture to those who hear the presentation. The presentation is about a person, not a list of problems. We must include and address the information about depression, foster care, and agitation, but leading with strengths respects the person as an individual human.

On a more directly practical front, if Jessica loves to draw, then we might see it as a warning sign if she were suddenly to stop drawing, or if she threw out her collection of sketchbooks.

Long-Term Risk Factors

Specific risk factors for suicide are discussed elsewhere in this book (see Chapter 4). The goal of the present section is to reflect on how knowledge about risk factors can inform clinical understanding and action.

The concept "risk factors" is taken from epidemiology and can be challenging to apply in clinical circumstances. The key is to remember that the "factors" are more than just statistical variables that predict risk; they are part of the "setting" to a person's story. Seen this way, they provide insights into what a person has been through, the challenges they have survived, and what kinds of burdens they might need help carrying.

Clinical Tip: Who Can You Tell Anything To?

When assessing strengths and protective factors, inquire about social support and connectedness. One particularly rich question to ask is: "Who can you tell anything to?" The answer can tell you (a) whether or not the person has one or more people they can trust and turn to, and (b) whether the person is willing and able to tell people about their inner life, and even about things that make them feel bad or ashamed about themselves.

Clinical considerations for eliciting information about enduring risk factors include:

Mental health history: It is not only about depression. Depression is often the first condition that comes to mind when clinicians think about suicide risk. However, other disorders, including anxiety, bipolar disorder, schizophrenia, and certain personality disorders, are also implicated. Many of these conditions can come with strong feelings of anxiety, urgency, and agitation – a feeling of being trapped and wanting to get out of one's own skin. This feeling can be particularly potent among youth. Understanding this dimension of a person's mental health condition can help in formulating an assessment that takes account of the felt experience of the individual.

6

Family history of suicide: If you don't ask, they might not tell. Having a family member who died by suicide means that a person has been exposed to suicide as an "option." They may see suicide as a viable response to pain and, consequently, may turn to it more readily. It is important to keep in mind that many families will not mention this history unless directly asked.

History of child maltreatment: Trauma-informed care is critical to suicide prevention. Research has shown associations between suicide attempts and all types of childhood abuse and neglect, with sexual and emotional abuse appearing to be particularly important in explaining suicidal behavior. Assessing and addressing these factors requires a trauma-informed approach.[1] Learning about a background of abuse can play a critical role in helping the clinician identify possible stressors that can be mitigated, as well as in safety planning that makes appropriate use of family resources.

Demographics: Avoid stereotypes; understand the experience. Risk factors can vary according to demographics, with different age groups, cultures, and sexual preferences, for example, all being associated with statistically different rates of suicide. Useful as this information might be, the primary reason for exploring and synthesizing demographic data is that this context is important for understanding **where an individual person is coming from** and for grasping how they, as a unique individual, might have been impacted by belonging to any of these groups.

Clinician Perspective

I worked in a pediatric primary care center for six years. Even though I was pretty detailed in putting together family histories, it wasn't until I started learning more about suicide risk that I began to directly and routinely ask about family history of suicide. When I did, I was shocked to find that so many of the children or parents I knew well had very close relatives who had died by suicide. Now, whenever I gather information, I'll ask something like, "In a family this large, has there been anybody who's died by suicide? How about any close friends?" That's one way to ask that might feel less stigmatizing.

Impulsivity and Self-Control, and Alcohol and Substance Misuse

Impulsivity is the tendency for a person to act without thinking, particularly in contexts in which their actions may put themselves or others in danger. People who have difficulty with impulse control can act quickly when they are frustrated or provoked. They are less likely to stop and think about how to moderate or restrain their reactions, and more likely to respond to situations without planning or considering the consequences of their actions. While there is not yet any consensus on how impulsivity works as a risk factor for suicide death, there is a correlation between impulsivity and suicide attempts.

Clinical Tip: Listen for the Experience Behind the Epidemiology

Information about the epidemiology of suicide is most useful in a clinical context if you ask about the individual experiences that might lie behind the numbers. For example, LGBTQ youth statistically have greater risk for suicidal ideation and behavior (see Chapter 16). But what do you do with these numbers when you are working with an individual? Rather than focus on statistical risk, let this knowledge prompt you to ask about the kind of experiences that might account for the epidemiology. For example, knowing that LGBTQ youth are at higher risk relative to the general population can lead us to ask about experiences that may play a role in that statistical risk, but which are specific to the individual, such as strains in family relationships, bullying, and sexual violence. Our goal in asking about long-term risk factors is not to categorize the person as a member of a group, but to use what we know about these groups to shed light on the individual case.

Alcohol and drug misuse clouds judgment and disinhibits risky behavior. Further, alcohol and drugs can restrict a person's ability to see that they have options available to them other than suicide to find a way out of their pain. When exploring a person's history of substance abuse, it is important to ask whether they were using drugs or alcohol when thinking about or attempting suicide in the past.

Drug and Alcohol Recovery: A Sensitive Period

While substance abuse can be an important factor for formulating a risk assessment, it is also important to remember that suicide risk can increase during recovery from dependence. Even if a person is being treated for a chemical dependency and has a good relapse prevention plan, it is still necessary to consider the risks that can come if a relapse does happen.

For both impulsivity and substance use, the most important clinical consideration is how these factors will affect the person's ability to follow through with crisis and safety plans. The efficacy of such plans will likely be diminished. This does not mean safety planning should not be used with persons who are highly impulsive or likely to use substances, but it does indicate a greater need to take other prevention measures, such as involvement of other support persons in plans and closer, more frequent follow-up and observation. These measures are covered in greater detail in Chapter 7.

● Dynamic Factors

Stressors and Precipitants: Listen for the Meaning

Most stressors that have been empirically linked to suicide (relationship disruptions, financial trouble, health concerns, etc.) are extremely common. The question then arises as to what makes an otherwise ordinary stressor become something that could trigger suicide. Leading theories of suicide[2–4] provide useful clues concerning what clinicians should ask about and listen for when hearing about a stressful life event.

Patient Perspectives

"After my suicide attempt, I knew I was losing my job. I felt humiliated, hopeless, uncertain. I never thought I would get better and have a job again. My job was central to my identity and gave me purpose and belonging … not to mention money to live on."

The key is to listen for the subjective meaning or consequence of the stressor. In particular, clinicians should listen for stressors that make the person feel:

- All alone, isolated
- Like a burden, having nothing to offer
- Socially defeated, humiliated
- Trapped

Settings: Pediatrics

If you work with families in the child welfare system, you will want to keep the welfare of parents in mind as well. In a 2017 study with over 10,000 mothers, mothers of children who had been removed from the home and taken into care had higher rates of suicide attempts and deaths than mothers who received services but did not have children taken into care.

Symptoms, Suffering, and Recent Changes

This key domain includes symptoms that are often found on diagnostic checklists. However, "symptoms" are generalized concepts rather than individual experiences, so the word "suffering" is also included in the framework here to reflect the more specific lived context of the individual person. Thinking about both symptoms **and** suffering can help remind the clinician that the assessment process is not just a box-ticking exercise but has a real human being at its center.

Hopelessness, feeling out of control, being more withdrawn, and feeling that there is no hope for improvement are the kinds of symptoms and suffering clinicians need to be particularly alert for. Knowing what might change for the worse for a specific person will also be central to suicide prevention planning.

It is important to note recent changes because they can help tell the clinician where a person is right now and can also provide some indication of where that person might be heading in the near future. In order to understand the dynamics of suicide risk, it is important to pay attention to whether symptoms and suffering are increasing or decreasing. Risk can only be assessed in a way that can usefully be applied if the assessment assists in understanding the trajectory of the individual's experiences.

Stressors and precipitants can also manifest as current symptoms and causes of suffering. Increases in anger, isolation, depression, and/or hopelessness can all translate into a sense of being demoralized about the future and into feelings of hopelessness about things ever getting better. Similarly, impulsivity and a person's sense that they lack self-control can lead to feelings of regret and to the suffering such feelings can bring.

Engagement and Reliability: Explicitly and Honestly Assess the Person's Ability to Engage with Services and Reliably Report their Distress

When assessing the gathered data, it is important to consider the level of engagement between the clinician and the person being assessed. The individual's degree of openness, their relationship with the clinician, and the extent to which they engage with the process all impact the kind of support plans that can be developed. It is important to be honest in assessing engagement, as the likelihood that important information may not have been volunteered will contribute to future planning. Concluding that the person has not engaged openly is not a negative judgment on them. Often, systems are not set up in a way that optimizes engagement for those with suicide risk (systems may be unfriendly, hard to access, inconvenient, or expensive, for instance).

A related issue is the question of the degree to which a person's report has been honest, reliable, and credible. Tools for improving the fidelity of data gathered are discussed in this chapter under the heading "Interview Strategies and Techniques." However, even when using such tools, a clinician may still in some cases suspect that the information they have collected is incomplete or inaccurate. If there are reasons to believe that a person is downplaying or exaggerating any aspect of their thinking, their behavior, or the things that have happened or might happen to them in their lives, then this needs to be accounted for in the assessment. The person might, for instance, suffer from psychosis, or have cognitive challenges, or even just change their story a lot. They may be wary about communicating honestly if they believe this will have negative consequences for their relationships with family members. Including these factors in an assessment, and in the communication of this assessment to colleagues, provides an important aid in calibrating how to deal with the other information that has been gathered. Determining that a person's account is not reliable does not mean making a moral judgment about their character. It is simply a case of determining how to help them as effectively as possible.

D Detecting and Understanding Suicidal Ideation, Behavior, and Risk

Some people who are considering suicide will report this spontaneously, but many will not. This section will review standard and emerging methods for detecting and understanding suicidal ideation, behavior, and risk. Methods for gathering information pertinent to suicide risk fall under three headings:

- Structured screening and assessment tools
- Interview strategies and techniques
- Emerging methods for inferring risk

● **Structured Screening and Assessment Tools**

Routine suicide risk screening using structured assessment tools is becoming standard care in behavioral health settings and, increasingly, in general healthcare settings.[5,6,7] Screening usually involves asking patients a few brief standard questions, either orally or in written form.

Organizations that wish to initiate screening protocols face several key decisions.

a) **Which Screening Tool Will We Use?**

A partial list of brief screeners appears below along with sample items and key references. Research on and common practices for use with screening tools are constantly being updated.

When selecting a tool (see Appendix pp. 279–280 for instruments and tools), the key considerations that need to be taken into account are:

1. **Number of items**. In settings where multiple screens must occur, every second counts. In such contexts it may be best to consider shorter measures.

2. **Standalone suicide screen or part of a broader set of measures**. For contexts in which a screen for depression or other mental health issues is either already in place or desired, it might make sense to use suicide-related items that are integrated with a broader screen.

3. **Evidence in specific population and setting**. If there are published articles showing the use or acceptability of a measure in the setting for which a screen is being considered, this research can help guide decision making. For example, when choosing a screen for a substance use setting, it will be helpful to search for screening tools that have specifically been tested in this environment. It should be noted that for many populations and settings no such research will exist. When that is the case, the only recourse is to acknowledge this as a limitation and educate staff as to the limits.

4. **Patient and staff feedback**. While academic evidence of validity in a given setting is important, a screening program will be most effective if the people offering and receiving the screen feel comfortable with the questions.

b) Who Will Be Screened?

The most critical decision for any screening program is whether the program will be universal (screen everybody) or targeted (screen particular groups) based on some specific risk factor or set of factors. This can be a challenging decision. Universal screening is likely to identify more at-risk individuals, but it will also require more resources. There is near consensus in the field that individuals seen for behavioral health (mental health and substance use) conditions should all receive screening, whether in dedicated mental health or in general health settings. Momentum is growing for universal screening in primary healthcare and emergency department settings but support for universal screening in these contexts is not unanimous. In 2014, the US Preventive Services Task Force concluded that there is not yet enough evidence to recommend universal screening for suicide risk in primary care.[8] Emergency Department screening is also still an emerging practice. In both cases the main source of hesitation about universal screening is the shortage of time and referral resources available for addressing positive screens. The direction in which standard practice will move is not yet clear, but the judgment of the authors of this volume is that universal screening will and should become a norm in these settings within the next several years.

c) When and How Often?

Screening should generally be conducted at an initial meeting, when there are signs of distress or concerns expressed by others, and at some routine interval (e.g., annually). Generally, it is best to conduct screening early in a patient encounter in order to provide time to address any issues that might arise. Screening universally at very high frequencies, such as every visit, should be done with caution and specific training should be provided on how to provide a caring rationale. One qualitative study with a veteran population found that patients did not like being asked about suicidal thinking at every visit. Such questioning could seem intrusive, off-putting, and insincere, as well as distracting from their subjective concerns. There is, thus, a risk that overuse of screens might deter honest answers and genuine engagement.

d) By What Method Will Screening Be Conducted?

One important decision is whether screens will be conducted verbally by staff asking standardized questions or via a questionnaire (whether paper or electronic). Research has shown mixed results on the question of which approach is preferable. One study found high agreement between written and interviewer screening but greater disclosure of recent suicidal ideation on a paper form. While this decision is partly driven by the logistical and administrative requirements of healthcare providers, patient preferences should be taken into account – asking advice from patients treated in a given setting can be very informative regarding the approaches that will work best for a specific context.

e) How Will Staff Be Trained and Supported?

Screening is unlikely to be valid or helpful unless presented in a sensitive, open, and collaborative manner. In fact, screening could increase a feeling of isolation and stigma if patients perceive it to be a rote exercise rather than an invitation to open dialog. Staff are most likely to present and respond to screens productively if they feel confident and supported. We recommend that training for screeners include the provision of a broad understanding of the experience of the suicidal person and specific tactics for responding to different scenarios, such as hesitation or a positive screen. The collaboration skills presented in Chapter 5 are especially critical, as is having a complement of "mini-interventions" as described in Chapter 7. A well supported workforce is critical to accomplishing the goals of suicide prevention.

f) What Is the Protocol for Positive Screens?

The ultimate purpose of screening is to identify opportunities for prevention. Screening thus carries with it the responsibility to follow up on positive results. There are several aspects to consider in relation to dealing with positive screens:

- Timely review. All patient screens regarding suicide risk should be reviewed and addressed before the person leaves the current visit. If someone discloses suicidal ideation and there is no response to this disclosure, then there is a risk of making things worse, and the provider may also have a legal liability (see Chapter 11).
- Proper training, skills, and time need to be made available to ensure there is provision to discuss and further explore suicide concerns that arise.
- Plans for adjusting schedules. Positive results on a screen will unavoidably require additional time for follow-up, so it is important to make allowances and to make plans to adapt schedules when necessary. Different mechanisms will be available in different settings. For example, in primary care the easiest way to free up time to respond to a positive screen may be to reschedule routine patients for later in the day.

Clinician Perspective

Sometimes after a patient has disclosed suicidal ideation and plans to me on a routine screen, I have had to extend the visit to address risk. Aware that this would cause others to wait, I went to the waiting room and asked another patient if they would be willing to give some of their time so that I could address the emergency. This has happened more than once and I have not yet encountered a situation in which they have said no. In fact, many patients feel good about being able to do something to help another person.

● Interview Strategies and Techniques

Standardized screening tools are important for gathering relevant and useful information about suicidal thoughts, plans, and behavior. However, many people who are seriously considering or planning suicide will not disclose this fact on a screen. Research suggests that approximately a quarter of patients who attempted suicide within a week of a screen answered "not at all" to questions about the frequency of suicidal ideation.[9] Some people might feel ashamed of their thoughts or actions, seeing them as reflections of a personal weakness or failure. Others worry about the consequences of telling a medical professional, about the impact sharing this information might have on their job or their family. Many people fear that involuntary hospitalization could result from honest disclosure.

In light of this information, it is critical that clinicians develop skills for eliciting suicidal thoughts and plans through questioning and listening. A number of valuable person-centered techniques have been developed for detailed inquiry – strategies that encourage the person to talk openly and honestly, so that information gathered is as accurate as possible.

Chronological Assessment of Suicide Events

One of the most powerful in-depth interviewing tools is the Chronological Assessment of Suicide Events (CASE). This approach proceeds chronologically, starting by recording suicidal thoughts and events in the most distant past and moving incrementally up to the present day. Competency in the CASE approach requires specific training,[1] but the basic idea, which can be meaningfully applied by most professionals, is to help the person feel comfortable sharing information about the past, which they may perceive

---

[1] More information about the CASE approach and opportunities to learn it can be found at the developer's website: https://suicideassessment.com/

as "safer" to disclose than present thoughts and plans. Exploring the past and slowly moving forward allows the person to test the waters. How does it feel to reveal this? Does the professional react in a calm and sensitive manner? Having opened up about the past, the person at risk sometimes feels more comfortable sharing openly about present thoughts and feelings.

Validity Techniques

"Validity techniques" are ways of asking about suicidal thoughts that are designed to increase the validity of the information gathered. The following toolbox of validity techniques can help overcome reluctance to provide honest answers about suicidal ideation and behavior, and to support the gathering of accurate information (see Shea 1999 for a systematic treatment of these techniques).[10] These techniques build upon skilled and personalized engagement with a person (see Chapter 5) and can be used by anyone.

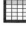 **Toolbox of validity techniques**

Technique name	Objective	What you do	What you say
Normalization	Open up the topic by letting the person know that such thoughts are not uncommon and that they are not unusual for having them.	Lead the person gently into the discussion of the topic, making it clear that many other people have, and have shared, similar thoughts and feelings, and have suffered in similar ways.	"Sometimes when people feel as depressed as you do, the idea of killing themselves crosses their mind. Have you had any thoughts like that?" "When people feel this bad, it's not unusual for them to think, "I would rather be dead than have to deal with this." Have you had any thoughts like this?"
Gentle Assumption	Makes it easier for the person to describe what they have thought and done if they do not first have to get past the hurdle of "admitting" their suicidal ideation or behavior.	Ask a question as if you are assuming that a particular thought or behavior has occurred instead of asking if it has occurred.	"What other ways have you thought of killing yourself?" [Rather than, "Have you thought of killing yourself in any other ways?"]

Symptom Amplification	Some people can have a tendency to amplify their symptoms, signaling how bad they are feeling by exaggerating their thoughts or actions. This can be a natural response, but when gathering data it is essential that as much of it be as accurate as possible. Setting limits on answers can help ensure that distortions are minimized.	Bypass tendencies to exaggerate and distort by setting upper limits to answers when you ask a question.	"On the days when you are feeling most suicidal, how much time do you spend thinking about killing yourself? 70%, 80%, 90% of the day?" "How many pills did you take … 50, 100, more than 100?"
Behavioral Incident	While it is important to provide outlets for emotions and to engage with the person's views, in gathering data about events it is vital to focus on collecting accurate information. When pursuing this particular goal, it is best to avoid clouding the reporting with anything that might obscure or derail the account.	Ask the person for specific facts, details, or thoughts concerning their suicidal ideation or behavior, with follow-up questions about what happened next. Stick to a factual account of the incident and avoid asking about opinions or impressions.	"Exactly how many pills did you take?" "Did you load the gun?" "What did you do then?"
Shame Attenuation	Offers a framework that allows the person to answer in the context of a ready-made explanation for thoughts or behaviors they might otherwise be ashamed of admitting. Creates an atmosphere in which it is acceptable to discuss such thoughts and behaviors.	Phrase questions in a way that allows for a positive response without the answer feeling like it is self-incriminating. Begin with a statement that sets a non-accusatory tone by framing the question in the context of a possible way of rationalizing the thought or behavior.	"With all the pain you have been experiencing, has it ever crossed your mind to kill yourself?" "You told me that you consider suicide a sin, but I'm wondering whether, with all the immense stress and pain you have experienced recently, did you ever have thoughts about suicide, even if only briefly?"

6

| Denial of the Specific (adults only) | Sometimes clients give blanket denials to generalized questions such as, "What other ways have you thought about killing yourself?" Asking specific questions makes it harder for the person to deny every item that is true for them than it would be to dismiss the whole category of questions in one go.

*This technique should not be used with children because of concerns about the impact of listing possible methods for suicide. | Ask a series of questions about specific methods of suicide, leading the person to individually confirm or deny each method. | "Have you thought about shooting yourself?"

"Have you thought about overdosing?"

"Have you thought about … ?" |

Asking Family Members and Other People

When significant risk is present and identified, it is standard practice to go beyond the person's self-report and to speak with family members and other support persons. These other people may not only serve as valuable sources of new information but can also provide an important means by which to validate information that has already been gathered.

But what if a patient does not want their family to provide information? Whenever possible, communication with family members should be negotiated collaboratively. However, most ethical and legal standards (including those enshrined in the USA in the Health Insurance Portability and Accountability Act 1996) allow for information exchange to take place without the patient's consent when suicide risk assessment or intervention may be required. These limits of confidentiality should be reviewed early with patients, ideally long before a crisis arises and the urgent need for communication comes up.

● **Emerging Approaches: Beyond Self-Report at Patient Visits**

Some people will not report ideation or plans even if they are asked. In response to this problem, research is currently ongoing to find new sources of information and to develop techniques that do not require self-reporting.

While not widely available, it is useful to consider these emerging approaches:

Implicit Association Tests (IAT).[11] Implicit Association Tests are a well-established method for identifying many kinds of hidden preferences and attitudes that the holder may themselves be unaware of. IATs have been applied in a variety of settings – such as revealing hidden prejudices or unspoken political beliefs – and have recently been tested for their use in uncovering suicidal intent. IATs involve showing the test subject a pair of terms – such as "good" and "bad" or "pleasant" and "unpleasant" – and then asking the subject to assign images or words to one group or the other. The speed at which individuals decide group membership can reveal implicit views, such as underlying prejudices, which would not be apparent from the classifications alone. For instance, a test subject might hold the **explicit** belief that men and women are equally competent in leadership roles, but be slower to associate images of women and female names with a positive leadership category, thus revealing an **implicit** bias. Suicide-related IATs have been tested using associations between the categories of "me" and "not me" and language associated with life and death. Initial results suggest that these tests can be helpful in identifying the likelihood of future suicide attempts in situations where suicidal ideation may not be apparent to the clinician, or even to the patient.

Ecological Momentary Assessment (EMA). EMA involves pinging people on phones or other devices to ask about suicidal thoughts or distress in "real time." This approach gets around one of the most significant limitations of self-report conducted in healthcare settings, which is that a health or behavioral healthcare encounter takes place in a supportive environment in which many day-to-day stressors, drivers (e.g., intoxication), and means for suicide are absent. EMA studies are also demonstrating how fluid suicidal ideation is, often showing large variation even within a single day.

Health record. Recent research has explored the potential for the application of big data analytics to databases of health records in order to identify individuals who fall into elevated statistical risk categories. A pioneering program – Recovery Engagement and Coordination for Health: Veteran's Enhanced Treatment (REACH VET) – developed for the US Department of Veterans Affairs is currently gathering data on effectiveness. The program uses machine learning to identify patterns in health records that are correlated with increased suicide risk, and then identifies veterans whose records include profiles that match these patterns. Proactive outreach by healthcare providers establishes contact with those with the highest risk and ensures that adequate treatment plans are in place. A 2018 study found that initial results of the REACH VET program showed promise.[12]

Social media. Research is currently ongoing to explore the possibility of training machine learning algorithms to explore big data sets from social media in order to identify posting patterns that may indicate suicide risk.

Sensors and other passive data collection. The combination of machine learning and big data also holds out the possibility of drawing signals from other data sets. With the increasing range of sensors built into homes, smartphones, and other devices come opportunities for testing whether sensor data can be used to predict suicide risk and flag concerns to healthcare providers. For example, one recent proof-of-concept study analyzed recorded sessions of conversations between spouses to seek to identify verbal cues that might be associated with increased suicide risk.[13] If this line of research proves fruitful, then microphones in phones or in homes, such as those built into Amazon's Echo system, could be used with the person's explicit permission to provide real-time detection of risk. Wearable electronic sensors similar to smartwatches can also be used to collect data on physical activity or heart rate (either at home or in inpatient facilities), while data on phone and internet use can potentially provide rich resources for mapping associations between risk and social contact.[14] Although not yet proven or in regular use, research in this area is progressing rapidly.[15,16]

 ### Synthesizing the Data for Communication and Action

● Prevention-Oriented Risk Formulation

The field of suicide prevention has struggled for a long time with the problem of how to summarize and synthesize the available information into a usable form that supports prevention. In the past, there has been a tendency to force the data into narrow categorical frameworks that are simple to work with but that miss the specific context of the patient's life, as well as the context within which the clinician meets and works with the patient. By contrast, the approach taken in this volume – prevention-oriented risk formulation[17] – seeks to integrate these contextual dimensions in a clinically useful way.

Prevention-oriented risk formulation has the following criteria:

1. **Contextually anchored.** Anchors risk summaries in the context of (a) the setting in which the person is currently supported, and (b) their own history.

2. **Sensitive to change.** Makes it possible to capture the fluid nature of suicide risk in the life of an individual and to explicitly state: **(a) how the person's current risk compares to risk at previous points in time, and (b) how risk might change in response to future events**.

3. **Actionable.** The risk formulation is framed in such a way as to **identify practical steps that can be taken to reduce risk**.

The core goal of prevention-oriented risk formulation is to promote communication and collaboration among professionals, patients, and families in order to reduce risk in the short and long term.

Risk Assessment Requires the Whole Team

Even if you never document a risk formulation for suicide in your role, it is useful to have a contextually anchored understanding of the nature of suicide risk so that you can understand how the formulation works and communicate with others about it. Everyone can understand that we want to think about the difficulties the person faces as an individual in their specific context, grounded in the situation they face and in this particular moment in time. Using this as our basis, we can then look forward in time to strengthen preventive factors and ask what might change and what we can do to mitigate problems that might arise.

Risk formulation consists of four elements:

- Risk status
- Risk state
- Available resources
- Foreseeable changes

Risk Status and Risk State

In formulating a risk assessment, clinicians can usefully distinguish between **Risk Status** and **Risk State**:

- **Risk Status is risk *compared to whom***, that is risk relative to others in a particular population or setting. In practical terms, when we speak of a person's risk status we refer to where that person "fits" into the bigger picture of others receiving services in the same setting or in a setting they might soon be transitioning into.
- **Risk State is risk *compared to when***, that is risk relative to the person themselves at other times. The point of reference for risk state is normally the person's baseline, but it can sometimes be another time period in their own history.

The concepts of risk status and risk state make it possible to connect a person's risk to their specific situation and environment, that is, to what is actually going on in their lives. By doing so, it becomes easier to find ways to help them deal with their unique circumstances.

Available Resources

Available resources are the strengths that patients and clinicians can draw on to support safety and treatment planning. Available resources might be **internal** (things the person has shown they can do if they start to feel worse) or **external** (someone they can rely on to act in specific ways during a crisis).

Settings: Youth

When working with youth, coping skills, trusted and trustworthy adults, and supportive staff and teachers at school are all available resources.

When identifying resources that are available to a person, a clinician might start with the strengths or protective factors the person has already mentioned. What is most important is that the things identified **should be specific** resources on which the individual can draw. For example, a known protective factor for suicide risk is having children in the home, but this will not necessarily be an available resource for a middle-aged man when he feels frantic or despairing about his finances. **Patient-specific** resources in this case might be strong coping skills, a supportive wife who knows about his treatment, or a friend at church with whom he prays every Thursday. Available resources need to be personal and they must have practical significance, because they provide key pillars around which to develop plans and responses.

A general rule of thumb is that it should be possible to **identify at least two available resources** for someone who is going to be served in an outpatient or community setting.

When Foreseeable Changes Need More Attention

Three aspects of the foreseeable changes will influence the level of contact and observation needed to support the person in the community:

- Are the changes likely?
- Will they happen soon?
- Will the change be visible to the team or to others who could inform them?

Depending upon your answers, a higher degree of care and observation may be necessary, possibly including hospital-based support.

Foreseeable Changes

Foreseeable changes are the kind of events that, if they were to happen, could quickly increase risk. These are the sort of situations that could lead to a crisis or could overwhelm someone and set them on the path to a downward spiral. Identifying foreseeable changes is vital for safety planning. Suicidal urges and ideation can be very fluid and can set in rapidly in response to significant events. By identifying them in advance, it becomes possible to put in place plans to help patients deal with them.

For example, if you are working with a mother whose children have been taken into protection, losing custody would be a foreseeable change that could have a dramatic negative impact on her state of mind. For a young LGBTQ person who is intending to come out to their parents, it would be valuable to formulate a response plan for situations such as the parents reacting negatively or even throwing the young person out of the home. In each case, by identifying a foreseeable change the clinician is able to work with the person to plan responses that can help minimize the impact of the change.

In identifying foreseeable changes, particular attention should be paid to changes that might lead the person to feel:

- out of control
- alone
- worthless or a burden
- humiliated
- trapped

These are all feelings that can precipitate or intensify suicidal ideation and urges.

Settings: Acute Services

We recommend identifying foreseeable changes for patients being discharged from acute services settings, whether or not they have previously identified suicide risk. A well-designed study published in 2016 examined 1.9 million hospital records and found that even those who had not been hospitalized for suicide risk were at greater risk for suicide after discharge from inpatient treatment.[18]

After identifying **at least two** events or changes that might significantly increase the risk of suicidal ideation or behavior, the next step is to then make specific and detailed plans for responding to each situation. If the person is able to work with clinicians to develop effective plans for each change (including a plan for addressing access to lethal means), this is a good indicator that their risk can be managed safely in a less restrictive environment, such as an outpatient setting.

The best way to address foreseeable changes is to develop plans in close cooperation with the at-risk person and their support persons. In some cases, the response plan might be obvious. One example of a foreseeable change is the person coming into contact with a situation that previously triggered a suicide attempt. In this case, the best plan may well be to avoid going to certain places in which that situation might arise, or meeting certain people who might lead them into such a situation. However, sometimes it will be harder to identify useful foreseeable changes and a degree of speculation – informed by what the person has said – may be required. Speculation of this sort may be considered to be a type of "disciplined intuition," combining information gathered from the person with educated guesswork.

Clinician Perspectives: Foreseeable Changes

Identifying foreseeable changes and developing plans for them is one thing that really lowers my blood pressure. One of the stresses I feel in conducting assessments, especially on discharge, is knowing how quickly my snapshot of risk can become outdated by changes in the person's life. I feel much better explicitly acknowledging the limitations of my assessment and demonstrating diligence by identifying what could happen. It helps me relax, care, and be effective.

Patient Perspectives: Foreseeable Changes

"When I was discharged from the hospital, I hadn't been seeing my current boyfriend, so my discharge safety planning didn't include anything about him. When my doctor first introduced me to the idea of "foreseeable changes," it was the part of the new planning process I related to the most. I thought, "What if we broke up? I need to update that 3-year-old plan!" It really changed my thinking about safety and recovery plans as being works in progress – they need to be updated."

Risk Stratification and Risk Formulation

6

The question of how best to summarize an individual's risk for suicide is a longstanding problem in the field of suicide prevention. Traditional approaches have tended to categorize people in terms of high, medium, and low risk. While the predictive validity of risk stratification has not been empirically demonstrated, stratification can be useful in developing services pathways, creating medical record alerts, and assigning or gaining access to enhanced care options. New ways of identifying and calculating suicide risk using technology may improve the predictive power of this style of risk formulation (see text box).

Clinically Applicable Frameworks and the Use of Emerging Risk Detection Technologies

New technologies are allowing increasingly sophisticated ways of making predictive risk assessments. "Machine learning" algorithms, for instance, can be taught to identify patterns associated with suicide risk and then set to mine vast quantities of data – such as medical record variables, brain states gathered via mobile EEG devices, and potentially even social media posts – to locate these patterns.

These new ways of calculating risk clearly have the potential to be useful. Knowing, for example, that someone has an 80% greater risk for attempting suicide in the next 30 days is helpful data that any clinician would want to know.

But the question remains:

Then what?

Whether risk is detected using a simplistic measure, such as a single self-report, or through an algorithmic assessment of tens of thousands of variables from a rich data bank, we still need clinically applicable tools and frameworks that let us think and communicate about the situation of the individual person. Without these, raw risk data can do little to help a person.

To whatever degree you make use of some form of stratification in your clinical setting, a prevention-oriented risk formulation offers significant benefits.

- Contextually anchoring a risk formulation relative to a population, setting, or a moment in the patient's life leads to a focus on the question of why this person's risk – here and now – is differentiated from that of another person, place, or time.

- Stratified risk categories conflate the person with their situation. Other conceptualizations have tried to get around this problem by distinguishing between chronic risk and acute risk.[19] While this distinction improves on earlier approaches, distinguishing between risk status and risk state takes this advance a step further by encouraging healthcare professionals to think about risk in terms of the situational reference points that are meaningful for the person's life.

- Risk stratification tends to under-identify serious concerns among people judged to be at "low risk." Distinguishing between risk status and risk state gives proper weight and attention to within-person deterioration. A person with few or no historical risk factors might have a lower risk status in comparison to the broader population. Nevertheless, they might, at the same time, also have a much higher risk state than at any previous time in their lives if they have just lost their job, suffered a bereavement, are feeling depressed and hopeless, and have begun to abuse street drugs. Such a person might be talking about killing themselves and may even have a means in mind.

- Communicating a risk assessment in this way helps to convey to others the domains of information that are driving the judgments about risk. Using these data allows clinicians to anchor their subjective judgments while also making the reasoning behind these judgments more transparent. When dealing with a patient who has been categorized according to the traditional method of stratification, the decision-making process behind that categorization can often seem like a black box. One of the benefits of the approach outlined here is that the reasoning is out in the open. This makes it much easier for other clinicians to see a patient who has been passed over to them as a unique individual, rather than as just belonging to a given category.

- An extended case example and risk formulation is provided online in our article about Prevention-Oriented Risk Formulation.[17]
  link.springer.com/article/10.1007/s40596-015-0434-6

Transparency

Clinician Perspective

"Use of a common and consistent language makes it easier to communicate with the person who is at risk. When all members of a professional team use the same structure to discuss progress and plans with the person at risk and their family members, it communicates stability and unity of purpose, and also makes what can be emotionally fraught communication easier to understand."

Patient Perspective

6

"Some of the technical language may need to be adjusted, but why not use the same framework to talk through my situation with me as you use to talk about me?"

KEY TAKEAWAYS

- Assessment is fundamentally about understanding a person, and empathy is an essential component in this process.

- The purpose of carrying out a risk formulation is not to categorize the person but to work out the best ways of helping them.

- Unless an effort is made to understand the situation in which a person finds themselves, it will not be possible to work with them to help find solutions for their specific difficulties.

- Risk is context dependent. The level of risk is not something in the person, but a combination of the individual and their situation. Understanding risk requires understanding how the individual sees themselves in relation to the world as they experience it.

- Risk is fluid over time. The same person might be relatively safe in the normal course of events but then be at significant risk if their circumstances change (a loved one dying, losing their job) or they come under new stressors.

- The context and fluidity of risk lead us to focus on asking "What should we do if something (internal or external) happens?" and "How can we plan an appropriate response?"

  Therefore, we need to identify:

  a. At least two changes in the person's context that could lead to things getting bad quickly (foreseeable changes).

  b. The resources that the person can marshal in crisis (available resources).

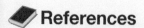

References

1   Substance Abuse and Mental Health Services Administration. (2014) Trauma Informed Care in Behavioral Health Services, Treatment Improvement Protocal (TIP) Series 57, HHS Publication No. (SMA) 13-4801, Rockville, MD, Substance Abuse and Mental Health Services Administration.

2   Joiner, T. (2007) *Why People Die by Suicide*. Cambridge, MA: Harvard University Press.

3   Van Orden, K. A., et al. (2010) The Interpersonal Theory of Suicide. *Psychol Rev*, 117(2): 575–600.

4   O'Connor, R. C., & Kirtley, O. G. (2018) The integrated motivational–volitional model of suicidal behaviour. *Philosophical Transactions of the Royal Society B: Biological Sciences*, 373(1754): 20170268.

5   Boudreaux, E. D., Camargo Jr, C. A., Arias, S. A., et al. (2016) Improving suicide risk screening and detection in the emergency department. *Am J Prev Med*, 50(4): 445–53.

6   Brahmbhatt, K., Kurtz, B. P., Afzal, K. I., et al. (2019) Suicide risk screening in pediatric hospitals: clinical pathways to address a global health crisis. *Psychosomatics*, 60(1): 1–9.

7   King C. A., Horwitz A., Czyz E., & Lindsay R. (2017) Suicide risk screening in healthcare settings: identifying males and females at risk. *J Clin Psychol Med Settings*, 24(1): 8–20. doi: 10.1007/s10880-017-9486-y

8   Gaynes, B. N., West, S. L., Ford, C. A., Frame, P., Klein, J., & Lohr, K. N. (2004) Screening for suicide risk in adults: a summary of the evidence for the US Preventive Services Task Force. *Annals of Internal Medicine*, 140(10): 822–35.

9   Simon, G., Rutter, C., Peterson, D., et al. (2013) Do PHQ depression questionnaires completed during outpatient visits predict subsequent suicide attempt or suicide death? *Psychiatr Serv*, 64(12): 1195–202. doi: 10.1176/appi.ps.201200587

10 Shea, S. C. (1999) *The Practical Art of Suicide Assessment: A Guide for Mental Health Professionals and Substance Abuse Counselors*. New York: John Wiley & Sons.

11 Nock, M. K., Park, J. M., Finn, C. T., et al. (2010) Measuring the suicidal mind: implicit cognition predicts suicidal behavior. *Psychological Science*, 21(4): 511–17. doi. org/10.1177/0956797610364762

12 Peterson, K., Anderson, J., & Bourne, D. (2018) Evidence Brief: Suicide Prevention in Veterans. Washington (DC): Department of Veterans Affairs (US). Available from: www.ncbi.nlm.nih.gov/books/NBK535971/.

13 Chakravarthula, S., Nasir, M., Tseng, S., et al. (2020) Automatic Prediction of Suicidal Risk in Military Couples Using Multimodal Interaction Cues from Couples Conversations. IEEE International Conference on Acoustics, Speech and Signal Processing (ICASSP), Barcelona, Spain, 2020: 6539-43, doi: 10.1109/ICASSP40776.2020.9053246

14 Kleiman, E., & Nock, M. (2018) Real-time assessment of suicidal thoughts and behaviors. *Current Opinion in Psychology*, 22: 33–7.

15 Kleiman, E. M., Glenn, C. R., & Liu, R. T. (2019) Real-time monitoring of suicide risk among adolescents: Potential barriers, possible solutions, and future directions. *Journal of Clinical Child & Adolescent Psychology*, 48(6): 934–46.

16 Torous, J., Larsen, M. E., Depp, C., et al. (2018) Smartphones, sensors, and machine learning to advance real-time prediction and interventions for suicide prevention: a review of current progress and next steps. *Current Psychiatry Reports*, 20(7): 51.

17   Pisani, A. R., Murrie, D. C., & Silverman, M. M. (2016) Reformulating suicide risk formulation: from prediction to prevention. *Academic Psychiatry*, 40(4): 623–29.

18   Olfson, M., Wall, M., Wang, S., et al. (2016) Short-term suicide risk after psychiatric hospital discharge. *JAMA Psychiatry*, 73(11): 1119–26.

19   Wortzel, H. S., Homaifar, B., Matarazzo, B., & Brenner, L. A. (2014) Therapeutic risk management of the suicidal patient: stratifying risk in terms of severity and temporality. *Journal of Psychiatric Practice*, 20(1): 63–67.

7 Responding to Suicide Risk

Ⓐ Introduction

Working with people at risk of suicide is rewarding, but difficult at times. When someone's life may be at risk, clinicians often feel nervous and concerned, both for the patient and for themselves. In Chapters 5 and 6 we looked at how to form a **connection** with an at-risk person and how to formulate an **assessment** of their risk relative to other groups and to themselves at other times. In this chapter we consider what constitutes a good **response** to this risk by suggesting four categories that can be used to organize the planning, implementation, and documentation of responses to suicide risk. Having a clear framework for what constitutes a solid response ensures consistent care and is comforting for patients, families, and providers.

- Providing treatment and mini-interventions to target drivers and promote recovery
- Engaging patients and support persons in meaningful plans for safety
- Adjusting contact/observation to support the least restrictive environment
- Seeking and documenting consultations with colleagues

Clinician Worries

"I love my job and it's incredibly rewarding, but it's also stressful at times. I worry. Primarily, I worry that a precious human being could lose their life and future. But I also worry about me. "Have I done enough? Can I go home and stop thinking about this?" And there's always part of me wondering what someone else is going to think if something bad happens and my work and documentation is reviewed."

 PRINCIPLES

- When risk changes, your response should change too.

- To inspire hope, think and talk beyond safety toward long-term health, recovery, and attaining personal goals.

- Whatever your role, in everyday practice you can draw on techniques and tactics used in evidence-based interventions.

- Be familiar with the locally used standardized Safety Planning Intervention form.

- Develop specific contingency plans for each foreseeable change identified during the Assess stage. In doing so, draw on the available resources identified during assessment.

- In addition to planning for addressing suicide risk in a crisis, it is critical to also develop plans to support long-term **recovery**.

- Make the environment safer for a person by collaborating with them on reducing their access to potential means of suicide, paying particular attention to their personal and culturally preferred means.

- Determine if there are unmet social or medical needs that might decrease risk if they are removed.

- Develop safety plans that employ contact and observation tools to support the individual in the least restrictive environment possible.

- Dealing with suicide risk can be hard for clinicians: consult with other team members and supervisors to gain new perspectives or to help relieve the pressures involved.

Treatments and Mini-Interventions to Address Drivers and Promote Recovery

This category is listed first to serve as a reminder that the goal in responding to suicide risk is ultimately the person's recovery, and not fire-fighting a sequence of crises.

Providing treatments means offering access to suicide-specific evidence-based psychotherapies and medications where they are available and appropriate.

Psychotherapies. There are now a number of powerful and creative therapeutic programs that have been tested with adults, and some have also been validated or used widely with adolescents. Therapists can become certified in these evidence-based treatments through specialized training programs, and new programs and research showing positive results are emerging all the time. Examples of such evidence-based therapies include:

- Cognitive Behavioral Therapy (CBT). Manualized, individual psychotherapy for persons who have recently attempted suicide. A number of different cognitive behavioral interventions have achieved good results with suicide attempt survivors and with military personnel.[1] These treatments have achieved 50%-60% reductions in suicide reattempts by targeting cognitive distortions that may motivate suicidal ideation and behavior.
- Dialectical Behavior Therapy (DBT). Manualized psychotherapies based on cognitive behavioral theory and techniques. DBT was initially developed to treat suicide risk in patients with borderline personality disorder. It targets suicidal behavior and other behaviors that contribute to suicide risk (e.g., reactive behaviors or behaviors that interfere with treatment or that destabilize the individual). Recent studies have shown that DBT can reduce attempts by 50%-70% when compared to a control group.[2]
- Collaborative Assessment and Management of Suicidality (CAMS). A therapeutic framework for assessment and treatment of suicidal ideation. The CAMS framework emphasizes the importance of collaboration with the patient and working with them to co-author their own safety plan, giving them agency throughout the process.

● Promising Brief Interventions

- Teachable Moments Brief Intervention.[3] This single-session intervention takes advantage of the period immediately following an attempt to make use of a particularly effective window for learning. The clinician explores with the patient what the attempt meant to them and patient and clinician work together to develop a stabilization plan.

- Motivational Interviewing.[4] The clinician interviews the patient in a way that leads them to reflect on their attempt and on the underlying motives. The goal of motivational interviewing is to shift motivation away from suicide and toward living and recovery by a nonjudgmental exploration of reasons for and against living. This inquiry allows patients to feel safe and free to explore their reasons for living and dying in a nondefensive manner, leading to increased openness to building on reasons for living.
- Attempted Suicide Short Intervention Program (ASSIP).[5] A person-centered brief intervention based around a narrative-based interview. The clinician helps the person tell the story of their suicide attempt in order to elicit the core information that is central to their own understanding of the events.

● Medications

A guide to medication therapy for suicide risk is provided in Chapter 9. To summarize the medications that have the most evidence for suicide risk reduction:

1. Lithium: One of the oldest treatments used in modern psychiatry, lithium has been underutilized in suicide prevention. Lithium has suicide preventive effects in the long-term treatment of both depression and bipolar mood disorders.
2. Clozapine: The first medication with a US Food and Drug Administration (FDA) indication for suicide risk reduction (for patients with schizophrenia). Still underutilized at present.
3. Ketamine: Rapid reduction of depressive symptoms and suicidal ideation. Esketamine is FDA-approved with an indication for Treatment-Resistant Depression and for adults with MDD who have suicidal ideation.
4. Antidepressants: Antidepressants can be used judiciously and effectively to address depression and anxiety. On a population level, suicide preventive effects are associated with increased population rates of antidepressant use.

Please see Chapter 9 and *Stahl's Essential Psychopharmacology Prescriber's Guide* for more detailed guidance.

Clinical Tip: Lithium and Mood Disorder

Consider lithium for patients with any mood disorder who may be at risk of suicide, and additionally if full remission has not been achieved. Also consider lithium for mood disorder patients, especially when suicide risk is present. Lithium should be utilized as a longer term approach, not a short-term antisuicidal agent. It is not clear how rapidly lithium works on suicide risk, given the methodological limitations of the data. Follow usual baseline laboratory and regular monitoring for renal, thyroid, and other metabolic side effects.

Chapter 9 also contains important caveats and considerations for using medication to address suicide risk.

Patient Perspective: Mini-Intervention

"I'm much more likely to trust someone, to stick with them for the next step, if they're honest with me – even if they're stumped. I'd rather you be speechless than have a bunch of easy answers to problems that seem unsolvable to me.

I've heard professionals say they worry about validating how bad I feel. But to me, someone actually acknowledging those feelings, how hard my situation is … and that I'm not crazy to want out … that's comforting. And I'm usually not hung up on them saying it the exact right way. I don't need you to be eloquent, just empathetic."

● Mini-Interventions

While evidence-based therapies are becoming more accessible, most clinical interactions with individuals at risk of suicide occur outside the structured bounds of an evidence-based psychotherapy session. To address this reality, clinicians can draw on tools and tactics that appear in manualized, evidence-based psychotherapies and apply them in other settings. Sometimes, being able to offer up an appropriate, simple, evidence-informed comment at just the right time can make a real difference.

The table below lists a catalog of useful mini-interventions that can be implemented very quickly and can have powerful effects when working with somebody who is struggling with suicidal ideation or behavior.

Mini-interventions: tactics, strategies, and phrases from evidence-based therapists that can be used anytime.

Mini-intervention	What you do	What you say	Objective
Moving next to the person	Move your chair to sit next to the person rather than across from them.	N/A	Creates a feeling of collaboration and the sense that someone is with the person in their experience.
Appropriate self-disclosure	When in doubt, tell the truth. If you are worried, say you are worried. Sometimes you will be left speechless when someone tells you they want to die or presents a horrific set of circumstances. If you do not know what to say, say that.	"This is really overwhelming, even for me, and I'm not the one going through it." Or "I really don't know what to say. I'm taking in how much you're going through, and I need a minute to process it."	Allows the person to see your human care and compassion; forms a bond of honesty; gives a place for genuine emotional reactions; gives you time to collect your thoughts.
Slow down and listen	Sometimes, the minute we hear "I want to kill myself," we think we have to drop everything and ask about intention, plans, means, etc. But often we can take a few minutes to slow things down and listen to the person say what they feel they want or need to say before getting back to our assessment agenda.	N/A	Helps understand what is upsetting the person and what is most important to them right now; helps build a bond by giving the person space to talk without imposing your thoughts.
Provide understandable models	Provide the person with a model to help them understand their suicidal thinking and to explain how such thoughts can develop.	See "Example models" 1 and 2. (See 'Highlight the desire behind the suicidal desire')	Help the person move away from seeing a suicide desire as something that must be acted on to seeing it as a tool that tries to meet a goal that could be met in other ways.

Mini-intervention	What you do	What you say	Objective
Example model 1: Highlight the desire behind the suicidal desire	This intervention involves suggesting, in any one of a number of possible ways, that there is a survival-oriented mechanism lying behind the suicidal desire. For example, you can explain to the person that suicidal thoughts can be triggered by a desire to escape pain and suffering, or by a desire to feel in control of a situation.	The underlying desire can be implied by asking questions, e.g., "Does thinking about dying ever help you feel more in control?" Alternatively, you can give a straightforward and simple explanation: "Some people say they actually feel a little better in a tough situation if they think they could escape by killing themselves. They don't really want to kill themselves. But they can't stand how they feel."	Drawing attention to the desire underlying suicidal thinking can help the patient see that dying may not be their *goal*. Once suicidal thoughts are understood as means to an end (i.e., reduce pain/suffering), it is easier to help someone see that they can achieve that end in other ways.
Example model 2: Contrast the tunnel vision of the suicidal mind with a vision of options	Explain to the person that some of the feelings they have and the way the world seems are a result of feeling suicidal. This is a mindset that can be changed.	"Our minds can play tricks on us sometimes. When you have felt really bad for a long time, you might start to think nothing could ever help. Does your mind ever trick you that way?"	Opens up the possibility of finding solutions other than suicide.
Radical empathy/ hope	Acknowledge the feelings of the person. It takes courage to empathize in this way, because many people fear they will sound as if they are validating the person's negative thoughts. It is important not to leave the discussion on this note but to end with an expression of hope and confidence in recovery.	**Empathy** "You're dealing with a lot. With all of that, I can understand how you'd be searching for some way out." **Hope** "Based on my own personal experience working with people in very dire situations, along with mountains of evidence on the effectiveness of treatment, I can see lots of ways that you can feel better. If you come in good faith, and we do our job, you can feel better."	The expression of radical empathy creates a safe environment for the person to bring up any degree of painful or frightening thoughts; assures them you will seek to understand their situation; and makes the person less defensive against statements of hope, as statements of hope are rarely accepted unless the person's suffering is acknowledged first. The simple expression of hope, especially grounded in personal experience and research evidence, can gently open up the possibility of other options for responding to a situation that feels inescapable.

D Meaningful Plans for Safety

Safety planning is a process, not a piece of paper. Thoughtful and person-specific plans for safety are an important element in any response to suicide concerns. Crisis and safety planning are a standard approach to treatment for individuals with mental health concerns. With proper engagement and connection with the person's own situation and motivations, safety plans can be an effective means of preventing suicide. If done improperly, safety planning can feel mechanical and impersonal, as if the person is "filling out a form" rather than rehearsing lifesaving steps.

Resources: Support Persons

Contingency plans almost always involve central support persons in the life of the person with suicide risk. But there are some cases in which the role of support persons becomes even more important. When dealing with youth, there will always be a vital role in contingency planning for parents or other responsible adults. The need to integrate support persons in planning can also be intensified when foreseeable changes involve substance use or when engagement or reliability is low.

Planning interventions starts with creating a **specific contingency plan** (see Figure 7.1) for each of the foreseeable changes identified as part of the **Assess** process (see Chapter 6). The goal in creating contingency plans is to understand exactly what the person, family member, and/or staff member should do if each of the foreseeable changes occurs. In developing these responses, it will often be essential to draw upon the **available resources** identified while formulating the initial risk assessment.

When time is short and risk is not immediate, the development of specific contingency plans for foreseeable changes – along with reducing access to potentially lethal means – can play an important role in promoting safety while more comprehensive treatment plans are being put in place. While not a substitute for a fully developed collaborative safety plan and treatment, creating a plan for each foreseeable change is an important first step for safety.

Figure 7.1 Simple Contingency Plan

Planning for Specific Changes or Events
(Foreseeable Changes)

As I take the next steps toward feeling better, what are two events or changes that could make me feel overwhelmed, suicidal, or put me into crisis?

1) _____

What can you or someone else do if this happens?

_____

2) _____

What can you or someone else do if that happens?

_____

● Safety Planning Intervention

The elements covered in the widely adopted Safety Planning Intervention are shown in Figure 7.2.

Figure 7.2 Contingency and safety planning[7]

The contingency plan provides a concrete plan for two specific changes that could occur. The broader safety plan covers broader warning signs, coping skills, and reduction of access to lethal means. © 2019 University of Rochester. Used with permission from licencee (SafeSide Prevention, LLC) .

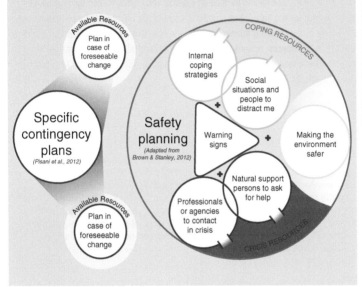

7

Example Prompting Questions (from ASSIP Manual)

- We have now seen how things developed, leading to a suicide attempt. What would be helpful in the long run to reduce the risk of future suicidal crises?
- How important do you think psychiatric treatment is?
- How important is medication?
- What would be your treatment goals for psychotherapy/counseling?

In Fig. 7.2, the various elements involved in safety planning and developing contingency plans have been grouped together using different colors. In the center are personal **Warning Signs** – the feelings or triggers that have led the person to suicidal crises in the past. **Coping Resources** are the steps a person at risk can take on their own without having to draw on external resources or even tell anyone else that they are feeling bad. These resources can include the person simply getting out of the house and distracting themselves with the company of other people. Finally, there are **Crisis Resources**, actions that involve the person telling others that they are in trouble. These resources are trusted friends or family, and professional supports who are available 24/7 to respond to a crisis.

Access to Lethal Means

Means Substitution Is Not the Norm

At a population level, policies and laws that reduce access to lethal means in public places, like putting barriers on bridges, have been some of the most successful suicide prevention strategies we have. When I first heard that bridge barriers could actually reduce suicides, it seemed odd to me. So what if there's a fence there? Can't the person take three steps back and get hit by a car? It turns out that this rarely happens. Most of the time when you reduce access to a particular preferred means people do not readily use another means – we rarely see what suicidologists call "means substitution."

Making the environment safer for a person with suicide risk by reducing access to potential means of suicide is critical. Short of hospitalization, it is impossible to create an environment in which there are no possible means by which a person can end their life. However, because most people will only be willing to use a limited range of lethal means, removing access to these specific "preferred" means can reduce risk.

Because of its direct and substantial impact on outcomes, means reduction should always be a high priority in safety planning. No matter how little time is available to create contingency and safety plans, this element is always central.

Statistics on the use of different lethal means for suicide show a great deal of variation by country and region, as well as by demographic and cultural group. While firearms are the most common method for suicide in the US, especially among adult men, suffocation is more common in the UK, New Zealand, and Australia. In some large cities, falling from tall structures is most common, while poisoning is more common in rural areas. In general terms, the availability of, and familiarity with, specific means are important factors.

Restricting access to some of these means can be harder than others due to their prevalence or scarcity. Similarly, reducing access to specific means may be more or less feasible depending on the particular care setting of the individual at risk.

Consistent with the person-centered approach to suicide prevention outlined above, the first priority for lethal means reduction is reducing access to any means that have been specifically identified by the at-risk individual. Clinicians can then focus on the means that provide the highest statistical risk based on the region and the population groups to which the person belongs. Some means are easier to address than others. For example, a support person can dispose of medication or monitor and confirm that disposal has taken place. Likewise with firearms, it is possible to ask direct and confirmable questions:

- What type of firearm(s) do you own?
- Where is it/they stored?
- Who will safely store the firearms?
- Is temporary storage outside the home possible? This is the most certain way to assure safety.

Everyday Lethal Means

Some lethal means that may be preferred in some regions or by certain demographic groups are simply "there" in the everyday environment (e.g., vehicles for asphyxiation, poisons in agricultural communities, bridges or clifftops). When addressing such means, there are no easy answers. Clinician creativity can be helpful, but the most important factor is paying attention to the individual and their needs. Often, the most important thing we can do to keep people safe in their environment is to focus on recovery and pay even more attention than usual to alleviating immediate suffering. While restricting access to lethal means is important when it can be done, ultimately what matters is the whole set of plans you develop, how these cohere, and how effectively they are followed up.

If the person is hospitalized, this planning needs to take place well in advance of their discharge, so that disposal or storage and verification takes place prior to the person returning home.

Firearms as Lethal Means

Because of the prevalence of firearm suicides and firearm ownership in the USA, almost all care standards require specifically addressing firearms access. Make sure you know your organization's policies, which are based on relevant local laws. If you do not already know, find out the rules about who can and cannot take temporary possession of a firearm, how this should be done, and under what conditions it can be returned to the individual.

Other means, such as jumping from high structures, are more difficult to manage. One way of dealing with this means might be to ensure that a person who lives out of town is accompanied into the city when they visit. Technological tools are also becoming available to help manage access to this means, with trials taking place involving altimeters that could provide warning if someone is ascending to considerable heights. However, tools such as these do not address chasms and bridges, nor do they help with the use of lower buildings. Limitations of this sort are why plans for positively improving a person's life in the long term will always be an essential part of preventing suicide.

If a person's preferred method of choice is always easily available, then increased monitoring and support networks are required. For example, a person whose method of choice is jumping from a structure may need to be accompanied by a family member when traveling to certain parts of cities. While no safety planning can make it impossible for a person to access certain lethal means, the goal is to present a barrier that will either make it harder or delay action long enough for the immediate suicidal urge to pass. We know that putting time and distance between a suicidal person and lethal means can be life saving.

Best practices for dealing with lethal means emphasize collaboration with the person and verification via a third party. A stress on voluntary restriction of access for a defined time period for the specific purpose of safety can also help to give the individual a sense of agency and participation in their own well-being.

● Support Persons

An important element in safety planning involves drawing on professional and personal support people who can provide resources in times of difficulty. These other people need to be clear about what their role requires of them, so it is important to integrate direct contact with third parties into planning and to help them develop the skills needed to motivate and engage with these people. If family members are not involved in safety planning, it is important that an explanation for this decision is included in the patient's documentation.

Plans concerning involvement with, and active awareness of the central people in someone's life should be central parts of care routines. For example, in the ABC Health system, mental health treatment plans are updated every 90 days. At this point, the system also requires that the safety plan and family support plan are updated as well. This provides an opportunity to hear about new potential resource individuals, as well as to learn about the disappearance of other people from a person's life. Instead of relying on chance, this sort of approach embeds shared plans and roles for supports in routine care.

Given the importance of collaborating with support persons, it will be useful to consider the attitudes, skills, and practices that facilitate productive engagement with a person's wider support network. One specific practice for engaging families around safety planning is the family support plan. Family support plans present the content of a person's safety plans from the point of view of one or more family members or other central support persons. The development of these plans involves taking each of the elements of a safety plan and reformulating them so that the support person knows exactly what they should do to provide support when needed. This might involve specifying tasks or timetables for monitoring the person or ensuring the removal of lethal means. But it can also involve explaining when and how they can connect with the professional care team if it looks to the support person that the safety plan may not be working as is intended.

For example, when using a Safety Planning Intervention, it is normal to identify "social strategies for distraction and support." For a young person, what is their parents' role in the plan? Is it to remind the person of steps they need to take? To drive them to take them? In an ideal world, these plans will have been developed with family input and involvement, but even when time or circumstances do not permit extensive upfront involvement, developing the support plan in more detail can be part of the follow-up routine.

● Limitations of Safety Planning

As the name implies, the Safety Planning Intervention[8] is focused on the important goal of safety in crisis. Planning for recovery – beyond safety in the moment – is equally important for offering hope to those struggling with mental health conditions, intense stressors, or other challenges that contribute to risk. We recommend attention to planning for and engagement in treatment, including what makes life meaningful and worth living for an individual. While safety planning is critical for helping to manage crises, the goal of a recovery-oriented approach is to help the person stabilize and get better in the long term. This means that it is important to do everything possible to make sure that the person returns for treatment and engages with the goal of recovery. In one evidence-based suicide prevention system, emphasis is placed in the safety plan on long-term measures that the individual can take and on asking the person non-threatening prompting questions about whether they value certain things. This approach – asking questions about what matters to the person – is also used in motivational interviewing to address suicidal ideation.[4]

Finally, while safety planning is important, it is not enough by itself. Studies showing the effectiveness of safety planning demonstrate its effectiveness delivered together with an assertive structured telephone follow-up.[4] At present, there is no conclusive evidence to support the claim that safety planning is effective by itself.[5] It is important to remember that safety planning is a key part of the overall approach but should not be used by itself as a shortcut or as a replacement for systematic efforts for follow-up and crisis support (discussed further in Chapter 8).

 ### Contact/Observation Frequency to Support the Least Restrictive Environment

A key component in responding to identified risk involves considering the frequency of contact and the level of observation and monitoring of the at-risk person. The goal here is to **support the individual in the least restrictive environment** that allows for appropriate monitoring and safety. These priorities can sometimes be difficult to balance, with the clinician needing to weigh the risks and benefits of available options against each other.

Contact and observation tools and techniques are not limited solely to hospital admissions. Hospitalization is an important option and can be the right choice in certain situations; safety plans need to include responses that are in proportion to the risk assessed. However, the most intensive and invasive option available should not be used as a default position. Instead, clinicians should begin by asking what plans and contact and monitoring arrangements can support safety in the least restrictive environment.

Common options to consider include:

● **More Contact**

   Is it possible for a member of the clinical team to see the person more often, even if only for a quick check-in? Wellness checks by mobile crisis or support teams are available in some areas, so it is important for clinicians to know what resources are available to them.

● **More People Involved**

   It is always worth considering whether it is possible to widen the individual's support network. For adults, this might include drawing on peer, family, professional, and, in certain cases, employer support. For youth, it might involve engaging a broader range of family members or including more members of the school team. Youth peers should not be given substantial responsibilities, but they can be encouraged to involve adults if they spot concerns.

● Better Monitoring

In many cases, it is simply not realistic for families to maintain a constant watch over their loved ones, especially for long periods. However, depending upon the situation and duration, some families are sufficiently organized, capable, and willing to keep a closer eye on an at-risk individual.

Patient Perspectives: Hospitalization

"Hospitalization can really help sometimes and for some people, but for other people or at other times it can hurt. Being in a hospital gives you a chance to rest, change medication, get quicker access to a psychiatrist, and have the peace of mind knowing that someone is checking on you every 15 minutes, or even more often. When you're scared of yourself, that's a comfort. But there are also things about the hospital that can make a person feel worse and even increase risk, like isolation, stigma, separation from family, and possible job or income loss. If you have a trusted therapist, you might not have access to them either while you are in hospital."

● Balancing Risks and Benefits

How can the benefits of pursuing less restrictive options be weighed against the risk involved when a youth or adult has expressed suicidal thinking, perhaps even with a method or general plan in mind? The key tools for making this determination are contingency and safety planning work. Unless someone is voicing immediate suicidal intent, the ability to develop a sound plan for each foreseeable change and to make the environment safer by reducing access to lethal means are valuable signs that the person can be safely managed in a less restrictive environment.

However, if it is not possible to develop sound plans to respond to foreseeable changes, then it is necessary to consider a higher level of care and observation. This is particularly the case if the changes that might rapidly increase risk are likely to happen, are unpredictable, or are unavoidable in the short term. Sometimes a higher level of care might also be considered if there is simply not enough time available to identify resources or to contact the people that are necessary to make or confirm the plans that have been developed.

Clinician Perspective: Feeling Responsible

It can be extremely daunting to decide that someone at risk of suicidal behavior should be sent home. It can feel like you are making a gamble with the person's life, and a natural response is worrying about being held responsible if something goes wrong. These feelings can be particularly intense if there are gray areas in the case.

The first thing to remember in these situations is that you are not alone. Important decisions like these should be made collaboratively with consultants and other members of your team. Drawing on a pool of expertise both improves outcomes for patients and provides you with professional support in difficult cases.

A second point to remember is that it is critical to document your thinking using a reliable framework. Not only does this help when communicating with other team members and with the person who is at risk, but it also gives you confidence that you know why you reached the decisions you did and provides a permanent record on which you can draw to remind yourself. When you are dealing with gray areas, it is a good idea to write down both what you decided for and what you decided against. What were the options that you rejected and why did you reject them? Get your thinking down on paper as soon as possible after decisions are made, while your thoughts are still fresh.

For instance: "Considered transport to emergency room, discussed this with family and team, but rejected for two reasons …" State your reasons for rejecting this course of action and then describe what you did do: treatment and mini-interventions, contingency and safety planning, increased contact and monitoring, and team discussion, consultation, and referral for unmet needs.

F Team Discussion, Consultation, Referral for Unmet Needs

Both patients and clinicians gain confidence and better outcomes when responsibilities are shared by groups of medical professionals working together as a team. Discussion and consultation can be helpful in a variety of circumstances.

Clinician Perspectives: Outlets

When lives are at risk it is very easy to get worked up or to become dismissive toward those who are not deemed "serious" cases. This is why one evidence-based psychotherapy for suicidal behavior, DBT, actually requires therapists to be in consultation groups – powerful feelings come up, and it is hard to do our job if we do not have healthy outlets for them.

Negative feelings – such as feeling angry, afraid, controlling, or distancing – can get in the way of connecting with a person. If a clinician is experiencing such feelings, talking to a supervisor or someone else on the team can help to provide ways to get past these difficulties.

Lived Experience Perspective

I've often been asked whether I think some people talk about suicide to get attention. The answer is "yes," I think they do. But in a recovery-oriented framework, that's the start not the end of the process. The key question isn't "Are they saying it for attention?" but "Why would they say that for attention?" I get why that's hard for a clinician to see in the moment, but when we focus on recovery dealing with these people matters as well.

7

These sorts of feelings can come up in a range of situations. For instance, it is easy to feel angry and frustrated when a safety plan has been developed in collaboration with the family, only to find that the family does not follow through. Similarly, sometimes it might seem like the person is only bringing up suicide because they are angry at medical staff or their family and they want to provoke a reaction. In cases such as these it can be hard to feel empathy for the person or to achieve any meaningful connection. These kinds of negative responses are natural, but they can also get in the way of clinical work. For this reason, it is vital to reach out to colleagues in order to help process such feelings and to move beyond them.

We recommend that teams include individuals with lived experience (see Chapter 10 for more on the role of lived experience in systemic suicide prevention efforts). These people, who have personal experience of suicidal thoughts and behavior, are a valuable resource and can help refocus clinicians on what is important – the person who is in distress and at risk. Talking with someone who can offer insights into the perspective of the patient can also be helpful in finding ways to connect.

Another situation that warrants consultation with team members is when a clinician begins to feel hopeless about a person. Hopelessness can spread quickly from patient to clinician, and it is critical that such feelings do not flow back from the clinician and reinforce the patient's own views. One signal that feelings of hopelessness have set in is an inability to think of any available resources or reasons for the person to live. It can be quite normal for a clinician to find themselves thinking that they too might seek to die if they were in the same position as the patient. When such thoughts do manifest, there is an obligation on clinicians to talk these feelings out with team-mates, a supervisor, or their own therapist. By drawing on others, it is possible to acquire new perspectives and to regain hope.

Clinician Perspective

Whether you're working in a large agency or in solo practice, finding the time to discuss risky situations is important, even if it can be tough to fit into an already busy schedule. For me, it is a matter of professional survival. I can't do this work alone. Two bits of advice about finding the time. First, use a framework for these discussions. If you memorize a consistent structured approach to summarizing information, you'll be faster than if you tell the story a new way every time. Second, be OK with "quick." A quick call or conversation can go a long way. Follow it up with a short note – one sentence or phrase is better than nothing at all.

Finally, in cases in which a clinician is extremely worried about a patient, it is particularly important to document in the record discussions with team leaders, supervisors, and consultants (including their names). In part, this is a protective move as it increases the clinician's confidence in their own work knowing that colleagues will support the decisions taken if needed later. But the most important reasons to consult with leaders is that they are often able to provide valuable insights and useful ideas.

● Referrals for Unmet Needs

Determining what referrals are needed and when is not simply a matter of finding the appropriate treatments for symptoms of depression, anxiety, substance abuse, or other behavioral health issues. While referrals of this type can be important, and should be made when needed, responding to suicide risk also involves making referrals that can help mitigate the stressors and foreseeable changes that were identified while **assessing** the person.

For example, a person might be talking about suicide as a result of despair about their poor health. This person may need a referral for an untreated medical condition or a follow-up on an existing condition that is not being managed. If one of the foreseeable changes identified is that the individual might be evicted, they may need a referral to deal with housing instability. Similarly, for a student whose struggles to keep up in class have been a stressor that led to a suicide attempt, a foreseeable change might be that they fail their classes. This person might need help finding tutoring or need an assessment for challenges they are having with learning. As with everything, document any referrals you make as part of the suicide prevention plan, and follow up to see if a person makes use of those referrals.

KEY TAKEAWAYS

- Evidence-based suicide-specific treatments should be offered whenever feasible.

- Strategies, tactics, and phrases used in evidence-based treatment can be used as mini-interventions in a variety of settings and roles.

- Collaboratively developing a meaningful plan for safety is perhaps the most important step that can be taken to preserve life. Contingency plans should be developed for **all foreseeable changes** that may increase risk.

- Removing or reducing access to lethal means may be the most important prevention step. Work with family and other support persons to achieve this goal.

- Responses to risk should support the at-risk person in the least restrictive environment possible. Involuntary hospitalization has risks as well as possible benefits.

- Safety Planning is a critical part of caring for at-risk patients but isn't sufficient on its own. Plans should include treatment engagement and steps to promote long-term recovery.

- Work with individuals at risk for suicide shouldn't be done in isolation. Consultation with colleagues and referral to address unmet needs are critical to a safe and effective approach.

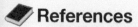 References

1   Rudd, M., Bryan, C., Wertenberger, E., et al. (2015) Brief cognitive-behavioral therapy effects on post-treatment suicide attempts in a military sample: results of a randomized clinical trial with 2-year follow-up. *Am J Psychiatry*, 5: 172. pubmed.ncbi.nlm.nih.gov/25677353/

2   Linehan, M. M., Comtois, K. A., Murray, A. M., et al. (2006) Two-year randomized controlled trial and follow-up of dialectical behavior therapy vs therapy by experts for suicidal behaviors and borderline personality disorder. *Arch Gen Psychiatry*, 63(7): 757–66. doi: 10.1001/archpsyc.63.7.757.

3   O'Connor, S. S., Mcclay, M. M., Choudhry, S., et al. (2020) Pilot randomized clinical trial of the Teachable Moment Brief Intervention for hospitalized suicide attempt survivors. *General Hospital Psychiatry*, 63: 111–18.

4   Britton, P., Conner, K., Chapman, B., & Maisto, S. (2019) Motivational interviewing to address suicidal ideation: A randomized controlled trial in veterans. *Suicide Life-Threat Behav*, 50(1): 233–48.

5   Gysin-Maillart, A., Schwab, S., Soravia, L., et al. (2016) A novel brief therapy for patients who attempt suicide: a 24-months follow-up randomized controlled study of the Attempted Suicide Short Intervention Program (ASSIP). *PLoS Med*, 13(3): e1001968.

6   Britton, P., Patrick, H., Wenzel, A., & Williams, G. (2011) Integrating motivational interviewing and self-determination theory with cognitive behavioral therapy to prevent suicide. *Cognitive and Behavioral Practice*, 18: 16–27. doi: 10.1016/j.cbpra.2009.06.004.

7   Pisani, A. R., Cross, W. F., West, J. C., Crean, H., Kay, A., & Caine, E. D. Brief video-based suicide prevention training for primary care. *Fam Med*, 53(2): 104–10.

8   Stanley, B., & Brown, G. K. (2012) Safety planning intervention: A brief intervention to mitigate suicide risk. *JAMA Psychiatry*, 75(9): 894–900. doi: 10.1001/jamapsychiatry.2018.1776

QUICK CHECK

A Introduction

The proportion of time a person spends in direct contact with a health professional is extremely small. We can make the most of our direct encounters by following best practices for connection and assessment and responding, as described in Chapters 5, 6, and 7. But ultimately, we must also consider how to extend the impact of our interventions beyond our healthcare environment into the lives and networks of the people we serve.

B PRINCIPLES

Extending care means thinking:

- Beyond the individual, to their network of family, friends, and other supports
- Beyond direct interactions within healthcare facilities
- Beyond the person's enrolment in a program or clinic or their episode of care

A set of key practices, service design, and systems structures that exemplify the extend mindset include ensuring:

- Input and clear roles for family and other supports

- Caring contacts to extend impact and intervention

- Proactive follow-up assessments and support

- Continuity and alternatives in suicide crisis care

- Warm hand-offs and continuity across systems

Patient Perspective

Words matter. As a patient, I don't want you to think of your job as "monitoring" or "transitioning" me. It feels more respectful to communicate that you and your organization understand that my life extends beyond when I'm with you, and that you're interested in how your assessments and responses fit, and extend into, my life.

C Input and Clear Roles for Family and Other Supports

● Planning with Families and Support Persons

The primary goal in involving support persons is to extend the core task of connection outwards. This means collaborating as early and as frequently as is possible with family, service providers, and other central supports around a shared goal of recovery.[1]

Chapter 7 emphasized the importance of developing safety plans that address the specific needs and situation of the person being cared for. A vital element in safety planning involves drawing on professional and personal support persons who can provide resources in times of difficulty. But these other people also need their own plans. In extending care, a key goal is to integrate contact with third parties into planning and to help them develop the skills needed to motivate and engage with these people – not as an afterthought but as central elements in the process.

Routinely Revisit Support Plans and Contacts

At ABC Health, mental health treatment plans are updated every 90 days. Coincident with this update, policy also requires updating contacts, persons involved in support plans, and their specific roles. If the person has declined contact with outside individuals, this decision is revisited.

Having a routine for updating and revisiting who is important and available in a person's life can make an enormous difference in the connection between clinician and patient and in the quality of care it is possible to deliver.

Awareness of the central people in an at-risk person's life, and the development of support plans in collaboration with them, should be core elements in care routines that are regularly updated. This provides an opportunity to hear about new potential resource individuals, as well as to learn about the disappearance of other individuals from a patient's life. Instead of relying on chance, making a concerted effort to stay abreast of a patient's evolving circumstances helps to embed shared plans and the roles of support persons in routine care.

Clinicians can draw on a range of practices, skills, and attitudes to facilitate productive engagement with a patient's wider support network.

● The Family Support Plan

One important practice for engaging families around safety planning is the development of a family support plan. Family support plans present the content of a patient's safety plans from the point of view of one or more family members or other central support persons. The development of these plans involves taking each of the elements of a personal safety plan and reformulating them so that the support person knows exactly what **they** should do to provide support when needed. This might involve ensuring the removal of lethal means or specifying tasks or timetables for monitoring the person they are supporting. But it can also involve explaining when and how they can connect with the professional care team if it looks to the support person that the safety plan may not be working as is intended.

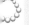

Clinical Tip: Updating Plans Together
Whenever a Safety Plan is updated, update the support plan as well. The two are integrally related and fit together hand in glove.

For example, a common element in safety planning[2] involves identifying social strategies for distraction and support. In the case of a young person, an important element in developing such strategies would be to determine what role their parents would play (e.g., reminding the young person of steps they need to take, or driving them toward certain behaviors or goals). In an ideal world, these plans will have been developed with family input and involvement, but even when time or circumstances do not permit extensive upfront involvement, developing a family support plan over time should be part of routine care.

Youth Special Focus: Availability of Alcohol

In the USA, alcohol is often implicated in youth suicide, with some studies suggesting it may even be involved in the majority of cases. Alcohol can play a role in disinhibiting suicidal behavior even for young people who have not previously abused alcohol or other substances. For these reasons, educating parents about securing alcohol is a top priority. Families can often misdirect their safety planning toward objects such as sharp kitchen utensils (a rarely used means of suicide) while ignoring open liquor cabinets or fridges of beer in the basement. Many safety planning documents for youth do not explicitly address alcohol in the home, so it might be up to you to add this element to your routine practice.

● Meeting Common Challenges in Working with Family

The challenges to involving family members in safety planning can differ significantly across care settings.

In youth-serving settings, approaching family members as potential assets and involving them at every step of the way is second nature. Thinking in terms of family systems is part of the job, so suicide risk should be approached in the same way. In acute services, by contrast, getting families involved is often difficult. Most inpatient hospitals have mechanisms for connecting with families, but it can be hard to involve them in a meaningful way unless family members are quick to respond, highly cooperative, and eager. Even when family members are keen to help, the pace of inpatient care and the need to stabilize and discharge patients quickly make it difficult to engage with family at a deep level.

Health and behavioral health settings fall somewhere in between. Professionals in these areas generally welcome family involvement, and it may even be a requirement when youth or vulnerable individuals at risk for suicide are involved. However, barriers can still arise in dealing with the broader care team, with collaborating providers, and sometimes from the person themselves.

There is no "silver bullet" solution to these challenges. What is important is to cultivate a mindset that treats extending care beyond individuals, episodes, and institutions as a standard. In developing such a mindset, it will be useful to consider a number of common barriers and to reflect on potential methods for overcoming them.

1. The first challenge is to recognize that **family members struggle as well**, and that they are not always equipped to help or easy to get along with. Making family members part of the team is an attractive ideal, but sometimes

the reality is that a family member's own struggles make them unavailable or even counterproductive.

2. The second challenge is that **some youth and adults do not want their families – or anyone else – involved and informed about their situation or care**. These two challenges can feel particularly difficult to navigate in certain cases, as when there is a legal requirement to inform and involve family.

Three basic principles provide invaluable starting points in these situations:

- Assume good intentions
- Widen the circle
- Widen the options

Clinician Perspective

When I'm invited to consult in situations with very severe suicide risk, it often happens that family members are described to me in a very negative light. It is natural for staff to feel angry when it seems like parents or other family members are working against the goals the care team is striving toward. One strategy that has helped me is to ask staff members to make a family tree-or genogram showing at least one generation above the "difficult" family member. We almost always find the same thing – significant levels of trauma. The recognition that the family member has their own suffering – and simply coming to know them a little more as an individual rather than an obstacle – makes all of us begin to soften a bit. When you can see that these challenging behaviors developed for understandable reasons, it can make the behaviors easier to work with and around.

Assuming that family members have good intentions may sound obvious, but it often takes commitment and effort. When family members present challenges, it helps to remember that nobody chooses to be disorganized, socially difficult, or drug addicted. Similarly, challenging or confrontational interaction styles are usually manifestations of a misdirected effort to have fundamental needs met. Once a positive mindset toward family members has been established, it is then possible to work together to find strengths and to capitalize on what they can offer to the process, rather than focusing on what they lack.

Assuming good intentions does not mean shying away from real family issues, as these can be important to tackle for someone at risk of suicide. Developing a set of feasible, acceptable, and convenient options for addressing structural and relational problems in the family will often be an important part of planning.

Clinical Tip: Uncovering Support Persons

Prompting questions can be used to help uncover support persons who might not be immediately obvious. A young person could be asked:

"Think about your bigger family – people you don't live with or maybe you don't even see very often. Who's someone you look up to or like to be around, or you think is cool?"

Widening the circle means thinking beyond immediate family in a way that takes in extended family members, friends, and others who are "like family" to the person. There is almost always at least one person in this extended family group who is available to be there when needed and who the person can trust. Uncovering who that person is sometimes takes work and may require prompting, but the process is worthwhile. It is just as important to find out who **could** be involved as it is to know who is **currently** involved with the person on a regular basis. In cases where there are issues with immediate family, discovering that there is a compassionate and concerned more distant relative who might want to help can open up new planning possibilities.

For many people, and particularly for those who have moved far from their family base, friends become a new family. When talking with adults, it is always worth exploring whether friends can be invited in by giving them a role in the person's care transition. Often, just knowing that friends are available and willing to help can provide a great support.

Settings: Youth

Involving friends can be a more complicated issue for youth. Friends can be involved as supports – providing distraction, encouragement, and company, and involving adults when they spot trouble – but the general consensus in the field is that adolescent peers should not be given formal responsibility for monitoring their friends or be the first person they reach out to if they are thinking about suicide. Nevertheless, young people tend to disclose their distress to peers often as a first or only disclosure, so direct communication between a care team and a person's friends can be helpful. With the youth present, and with permission from parents or guardians (for both the youth at risk and the friend), a team can talk with friends and explicitly discuss their role.

Another important consideration when working with minors is that it is essential to discuss the limits of confidentiality with them at the very beginning of the process, and long before crisis or concerns about confidentiality come up. This should be a standard element when a carer introduces themselves and their role. If it is necessary to involve parents when the minor does not want them involved, they should know from the start that this is part of the carer's role so that it does not seem to be a betrayal if it happens.

Sometimes, even when dealing with a wider circle including extended family and friends, there may still be challenges to involvement. This can include the fact that the involvement of family, friends, or even professionals is not always welcomed by the person themselves. At other times, it might be useful to involve a professional from another organization but they are not willing to play their part. In such circumstances, the next step is to **widen the options** for how input and involvement occurs.

Widening the options means taking a creative and flexible approach to family and professional involvement for the person at risk for suicide. Some things are not negotiable. For example, when a youth is expressing suicidal ideation, it is an obligation to inform their legal guardians and to document communication with them about safety plans. But even in such legally required circumstances, there is often room to be creative regarding how this involvement occurs.

Widening the options

Action	What you can do	What you can say	Objective
Offer one-way communication	Ask them if they would allow you to contact someone who may have useful information in order to hear what they have to say, but without discussing the at-risk person's situation, planning, or treatment.	"I wonder if we could start by getting your permission for me to listen to their ideas, but not share information about you."	When the youth or adult at risk is worried about sharing private information, gaining permission to just receive information from a family member or another professional can be helpful.
Propose an experiment	Explain to them that worries about how a family member might respond are both common and reasonable, while raising the possibility that they can also sometimes lead to valuable outcomes. Suggest that a good way forward is to test the idea in an experimental way before deciding how to proceed.	"You have the feeling that involving your brother wouldn't go well, that he won't understand or won't care. Could we do an experiment – have one conversation with him on the phone and decide after we see how it goes?" Or, "Why don't we call him, set our timers for five minutes, and check how you're feeling when the timer goes off?"	Validate the person's concern that a discussion with family might not go well while opening up the possibility that the results may be pleasantly surprising.

Action	What you can do	What you can say	Objective
Give control where you can: who, how, and how much	For example, share information only in the person's presence, or agree in advance what information will and will not be discussed.	"These conversations are about you. We need to have other people in your life involved but how we do that is up to you."	Gain the person's trust by giving them control over the circumstances of sharing information or involving others.

Notice that these techniques all involve getting an initial "foot in the door" in order to allow the most essential communication to take place. Once the door is open a crack, the eventual goal is to have broader involvement and communication.

● Contact with Other Professionals

Many of the principles that apply when extending care outwards to take in families also apply when involving other professionals in caring for a person.

It is important to remember that at-risk people often have contact with a number of other professionals in the healthcare system. This in itself provides a valuable resource that should be drawn upon in planning. These contacts can act to multiply the effectiveness of interventions, by using them as opportunities to reinforce plans and improve monitoring, for instance. Collaborating with other professionals in this way also multiplies the number of opportunities for a moment of need to coincide with some form of professional healthcare contact beyond the limited schedule of meetings with a specific professional who is focused primarily on treating suicide risk.

It is a professional courtesy, as well as good practice, to make sure that other professionals are informed if they are given a role in a person's support plan. For instance, if an element in the safety plan requires the individual to contact their primary care clinician under certain circumstances, then it is important to let the clinician know what to expect from the patient and what actions they can usefully take. Collaboration requires communication, and it will only be possible to leverage opportunities effectively if efforts are made to reach out and involve as many people as possible.

Sharing Safety Plans and Risk Data

In an electronic health record, patient notes are often walled off in a separate section rather than being available to everyone who accesses the record. However, certain elements of the safety plan should be accessible across the system, and plans should be put in place for sharing across systems using secure electronic Health Information Exchanges. A Health Information Exchange service allows care teams to share records across institutions and practices, making patient information available where and when it is needed to provide the best quality care.

Patients need to be fully informed about what data will be shared and with whom, as well as about their rights to confidentiality. One vital exception to all limitations on information sharing occurs in cases in which information is being received or provided in order to assess or intervene with **immediate** suicide risk. In such cases, confidentiality must come second to the person's safety and the preservation of their life.

8

D Non-Demand Caring Contacts

Non-demand caring contacts are brief communications that are usually delivered at regular intervals after care transitions or when someone is no longer enrolled in a program or facility. Contact is normally made by letter or text and places no demands on the person either to generate the contact or to respond to it.

Caring Contact Sample Letter

Dear Mr. Reynolds,

It has been some time since you were here at the hospital, and we hope things are going well for you. If you wish to drop us a note we would be glad to hear from you.

This practice originated in outreach to patients who had been hospitalized for depression or suicide risk but then declined ongoing care. In the seminal study of non-demand caring contacts,[3] out of 3,005 hospitalized patients, 843 (28%) did not engage in after-care. Patients who did not engage were randomly assigned to two groups. The first group received a post-discharge caring letter four to five times a year for five years while the control group did not. The group that received letters was found to have a significantly lower suicide rate for the first two years following the letters, and their improved outcomes continued for many years after. While the differences in outcomes gradually diminished, they remained detectable until the fourteenth year after discharge. The letter sent to the active group was just two sentences long, but those two brief sentences had a measurable lifesaving impact. Other programs have since expanded on this approach and have developed different ways in which caring contacts can be implemented,[4,5] including using postcards[6] and digital media such as text message.[7] However, the key elements remain the same: 1) letting the person know that they have not been forgotten, that they are not on their own, and that there are resources they can draw on; and 2) communicating these facts in a way that requires no action by the person at risk. Results across studies of different types of caring contact have not been identical, so more research is needed to determine exactly what it is that makes such contacts more or less effective. However, there is consensus among researchers that non-demand caring contacts have the potential to reduce suicide in a cost- and time-effective way.

In addition to post-discharge, caring contacts can be used to maintain contact when a person transitions from one program to another, or for youth whose cases move on to be handled by other organizations or agencies, possibly due to entering adulthood. By providing a link back to earlier episodes of care, the person is encouraged to feel that they are not simply being shuffled from one impersonal context to another, but that people who have cared for them in the past continue to do so.

Settings: Behavioral Health

Since the publication of the first research study into caring contacts, many inpatient psychiatric programs have begun to build post-discharge contacts into their general care. Patients who have been hospitalized have greater risk for suicide and, despite best intentions, many of these patients do not receive long-term follow-up care. While not a substitute for long-term care, caring contacts can help bridge this gap.

The timing and logistics for sending a non-demand caring contact to an at-risk patient will differ depending on the setting in which they were cared for and the context to which they are transitioning. In some cases, a deeper ongoing relationship will be maintained, as is typical in primary care, while in others there is a clear discharge point, as when a behavioral health hospital stay ends. But regardless of context, a caring letter signals ongoing concern **for** the person **from a person**. This communicates an attitude toward their care that may differ from experiences they have had in the past.

Caring contacts will ideally be triggered automatically at a systems level. The cost and effort involved in sending individual contacts in this way is very low, but setting up the system may initially require more significant resources. One common approach is to make use of event-based notifications in electronic health records. These can trigger responses whenever a patient experiences a given care event (e.g., notifying a primary care clinician when a patient is hospitalized). The sophistication of such systems is increasing rapidly, and many can now be set to include time-based triggers for patient communications. Use of these triggers can allow for a caring letter to be prepared and routed for signing by someone in the person's provider group a month after discharge, for instance, or any time the patient has not been in contact for 60 consecutive days. Depending on the sophistication of the available system, other sets of more customized rules may also be possible.

 Proactive Follow-up Assessments and Support

The use of follow-up assessments and support and the provision of access to crisis services is critical to support patients in transitions. High rates of suicide after psychiatric hospitalization[1] highlight the need for strong, proactive follow-up support during this and other care transitions.

8

Structured follow-up involves assertive outreach to individuals who are no longer in care settings. The goal here is closer contact and observation using protocols for planned telephone follow-up assessments. Research on this approach has primarily focused on people seen for suicidal thoughts and behavior in emergency settings. In one study, suicidal patients received a Safety Planning Intervention during their Emergency Department visit.[9] They then received structured telephone follow-up calls twice in the subsequent six months. During those calls, researchers reassessed suicide risk, reviewed and revised the safety plan, and encouraged treatment engagement. Use of the safety plan **plus** structured telephone follow-up was associated with a reduction in suicidal behavior and increased treatment engagement when compared to former emergency department patients who had not received the telephone intervention.

 Continuity and Alternatives in Suicide Crisis Care

Clinical Tip

When you give a person your on-call number and the number of a crisis line as part of your safety planning, have them enter them into their phone while you are present. This both ensures that they have these numbers and helps substantiate the sense of connection with you and the health system you are part of.

Local and national **crisis centers** can also play a significant role in extending contact and support, and in supporting the least restrictive environment possible for a person. It is now the standard of care everywhere to provide at-risk persons with contact information for telephone, text, or other crisis lines[10-12] that offer 24/7 on-demand interventions. These points of contact should include ways to reach on-call providers **within** the person's particular health system **as well as** access to third-party crisis care. There are currently ongoing efforts in various parts of the world to create better links between health systems and third-party providers, so as to enable crisis center resources to be integrated into local healthcare systems (see Chapter 10). The degree of integration varies from place to place, so care should be taken to check what resources are available for specific individuals.

 Warm Hand-Offs and Continuity Across Systems

Increasingly, the baseline standard of care in transitions and referrals for people with suicide risk is to make **warm hand-offs,** in which the referring health or behavioral health provider contacts the receiving provider to help make an appointment and, later, to check if the person arrived as scheduled. Paradigms are now shifting from a focus on making a referral to a focus on making sure that the referral works. Both making the referral and the administrative routines required for following up draw on specific skills.

In primary care and other healthcare settings, there are specific things clinicians can do to make behavioral health referrals stick. Regardless of whether the referral is to a co-located provider or to a specialist located far away, a skillful referral to address suicide concerns involves:

- Communicating to the referred person that you are expanding the team, not sending them away.
- Talking with the receiving provider in front of the patient. In co-located settings, this is ideally an in-person introduction. When referring out, it can involve making a phone call in front of the patient.
- Conveying confidence in the helpfulness of behavioral health treatment and in the abilities of the specific receiving provider.
- Expressing a willingness to problem-solve if the referral does not work out or if the match does not seem right. This creates the realistic expectation that referrals may or may not work out on the first attempt. It also side-steps the barriers that may arise if a person does not take up a referral, which can sometimes present an obstacle that deters them from returning for treatment.

By validating the person's choices, and not presenting a referral as the end point, individuals are encouraged to come back and see what else might work.

As far as administration is concerned, established relationships and a memorandum of understanding with select providers can be extremely helpful, as this foundation allows information and problem-solving to flow easily.

Pearl

If those making referrals **and** those receiving them seem like they are on the same page, the experience of moving on to the next provider gives a sense of connection, collaboration, and hope for recovery.

Where possible, referrals should be made to providers who share a common approach with the referrer. The "warmest" of warm hand-offs take place when the person experiences a continuity of consistent care across what feels like a coherent system and community.

8

KEY TAKEAWAYS

- Family support plans complement safety plans by communicating and making explicit the roles that other people play.

- Widening the circle of involvement and support can be challenging. However, maintaining a commitment to this goal through persistent and routine revisiting can pay significant dividends.

- A simple letter after a person has left care reminding them of your availability is a powerful evidence-based intervention that can have lasting effects.

- Providing contact details for crisis care and options for continuing care can equip a person with tools that can help keep them safe and make them feel in control.

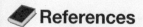
References

1   Asarnow, J. R., Berk, M., Hughes, J. L., & Anderson, N. L. (2015) The SAFETY Program: a treatment-development trial of a cognitive-behavioral family treatment for adolescent suicide attempters. *Journal of Clinical Child & Adolescent Psychology*, 44(1): 194–203.

2   Stanley, B., & Brown, G. K. (2012) Safety planning intervention: A brief intervention to mitigate suicide risk. *Cognitive and Behavioral Practice*, 19(2): 256–264.

3   Motto, J. A., & Bostrom, A. G. (2001) A randomized controlled trial of postcrisis suicide prevention. *Psychiatr Serv*, 52(6): 828–833.

4   Reger, M. A., Luxton, D. D., Tucker, R. P., et al. (2017) Implementation methods for the caring contacts suicide prevention intervention. *Professional Psychology: Research and Practice*, 48(5): 369–77.

5   Ammerman, B. A., Gebhardt, H. M., Lee, J. M., Tucker, R. P., Matarazzo, B. B., & Reger, M. A. (2020) Differential preferences for the Caring Contacts suicide prevention intervention based on patient characteristics. *Archives of Suicide Research*, 24(3): 1–12. pubmed.ncbi.nlm.nih.gov/31213148/

6   Carter, G. L., Clover, K., Whyte, I. M., Dawson, A. H., & D'Este, C. (2005) Postcards from the EDge project: randomised controlled trial of an intervention using postcards to reduce repetition of hospital treated deliberate self poisoning. *BMJ*, 331(7520): 805.

7   Comtois, K. A., Kerbrat, A. H., DeCou, C. R., et al. (2019) Effect of augmenting standard care for military personnel with brief caring text messages for suicide prevention: a randomized clinical trial. *JAMA Psychiatry*, 76(5): 474–83.

8   Chung, D., Ryan, C., Hadzi-Pavlovic, D., Singh, S., Stanton, C., & Large, M. (2017) Suicide rates after discharge from psychiatric facilities: A systematic review and meta-analysis. *JAMA Psychiatry*, 74(7): 694–702.

9   Stanley, B., Brown, G. K., Brenner, L. A., et al. (2018) Comparison of the safety planning intervention with follow-up vs usual care of suicidal patients treated in the emergency department. *JAMA Psychiatry*, 75(9): 894–900.

10 Gould, M. S., Lake, A. M., Munfakh, J. L., et al. (2019) Helping callers to the National Suicide Prevention Lifeline who are at imminent risk of suicide: evaluation of caller risk profiles and interventions implemented. *Suicide Life-Threat Behav*, 244: 16–20.

11 Gould, M. S., Lake, A. M., Galfalvy, H., et al. (2018) Follow-up with callers to the National Suicide Prevention Lifeline: Evaluation of callers' perceptions of care. *Suicide Life-Threat Behav*, 48(1): 75–86.

12 Shaw, FF-T., & Chiang, W-H. (2019) An evaluation of suicide prevention hotline results in Taiwan: caller profiles and the effect on emotional distress and suicide risk. *J Affect Disord*, 244: 16–20.

9

Use of Medications in Suicide Prevention

Ⓐ PRINCIPLES

- It important to stay grounded in the data related to medications in the context of treating patients at risk for suicide.

- These medication guidelines should be considered for more patients than just for those who are actively expressing suicidal ideation or plans, since longer term suicide risk can be improved with a comprehensive treatment plan that includes medications.

- This chapter aims to address any confusion that may still exist among the public and even among prescribers, about the relative harm and benefits related to medications and suicide prevention/risk.

- An overarching set of principles are presented to guide clinicians' decision making related to medication use when suicide risk is elevated.

- These principles include a framework that includes the clinical targets of both the patient's primary psychiatric condition(s), as well as suicide risk as a separate and appropriate target of clinical intervention.

- Medications such as lithium, clozapine, ketamine, and other medications with newer mechanisms of action with suicide risk-reducing potential, and antidepressants as a class are discussed in further detail with key clinical takeaways.

- The relationship with you as an ongoing health provider in the patient's life can be a powerfully protective factor for patients at risk for suicide. While discussing and/or prescribing medications, remember that your caring tone and compassionate communication, even during an otherwise more technical discussion of medications, can have a therapeutic effect.

B | **Overarching Approach to Medications for Patients with Suicide Risk**

● Medications Have a Role to Play in Preventing Suicide

To optimize outcomes with medications when caring for patients whose suicide risk has been identified, consider the following overarching principles:

1. **For which patients does this guidance apply?** These principles should be applied in clinical decision making for a broader group of patients than just those with expressed suicidal ideation. Suicide risk includes any patients with elevated risk, many of whom do not present with a chief complaint of suicidal ideation. Their risk may be identified by a recent suicide attempt, or by a family history of suicide along with current psychosocial stressors, or the patient facing a life transition or loss along with deterioration in clinical status. (See Suicide Risk Assessment in Chapter 6). At the broadest level, current clinical standards (including those of The Joint Commission which is based in the USA but accredits health systems in the USA and internationally) consider all patients being treated in behavioral healthcare settings (psychiatric inpatient and outpatient care, psychological therapy, substances use disorder treatment, etc.) as having potentially elevated suicide risk. In primary care and other non-behavioral health settings, any patient with a mental health concern or psychiatric condition (including substance use disorder) is considered appropriate for suicide screening. Thus, consideration of "patients at risk for suicide" should be broadened beyond just those with current ideation.

2. **When considering medications, discuss with the patient the risks and benefits on both sides**. Address the potential ramifications (risks and benefits) of not using medication, i.e., using non-pharmacological treatments or not treating the mental health condition, versus the risks and benefits of using medication, possibly in concert with therapy or another non-pharmacological treatment. Unaddressed severe major depressive disorder (TRD) for example, has known likely outcomes including disability, suffering, increased medical comorbidity, negative impacts on medical conditions such as cardiac, chronic

pain and autoimmune conditions, and an elevated risk of suicide by as much as seven times, as well as 50% increased risk in non-suicide mortality compared with non-depressed people or when depression is in remission.[1] In other words, the risks of not treating the condition or treating with only non-pharmacological modalities must be weighed against the risks of the treatment. And alternatives to a particular medication under consideration must also be discussed. This process of informed consent is good practice, and important to document from a medicolegal standpoint, as well as being truly useful for patients' understanding and engagement in their treatment. The same approach considering the risks and benefits of a particular medication in relationship to suicide risk and prevention can be utilized, as outlined in Figure 9.1.

Figure 9.1 Suicide-specific informed consent model

The same process of weighing risks and benefits of treatment versus not using the treatment can be applied to suicide risk, as we are accustomed to doing related to the outcomes of a psychiatric illness (or any health condition).

Risks (in Relation to Suicide) of Treatment	Benefits (for Reducing Suicide Risk) of Treatment
Risks (in Relation to Suicide) of not using this Treatment	Benefits (for Reducing Suicide Risk) of not using this Treatment

Alternatives to Treatment Under Consideration

3. **Optimize medication(s) for the primary psychiatric condition(s)**. Per usual practice, this should include a baseline evaluation/diagnosis/assessment of the mental health condition(s), education about condition, prognosis, and treatment, regular follow-up, monitoring of and adjusting for side effects, use of clinical assessment, scales and instruments as appropriate to track changes in symptoms and overall improvement, and adjusting the treatment plan including medication as necessary to maximize improvement. For depression, aim for full remission to every extent possible; consider medication dose

adjustment, augmentation strategies and referral to CBT or other forms of psychotherapy. Optimal results are often achieved with a combination of medications and therapy. Electroconvulsive therapy (ECT) and transcranial magnetic stimulation (rTMS has FDA approval for TRD) should be considered for treatment refractory patients with severe or psychotic depression and bipolar disorder. Both of these forms of treatment may also be helpful in reducing suicide risk.[2,3]

4. **Consider suicide risk as its own target of treatment**. This includes consideration of all treatments and interventions with evidence for suicide risk reducing potential. (See pp. 116 and 226 for psychotherapies with evidence for preventing suicide and remember safety planning as a brief intervention with risk-reducing potential.) In terms of medications, consider these medications which have the most evidence for suicide risk reduction:

    a. Lithium: One of the oldest treatments used in modern psychiatry, it has been and still is underutilized. Has suicide preventive effect in the long-term treatment of both depression and bipolar mood disorders.

    b. Clozapine: Until 2020 Clozapine was the only medication with an FDA indication mentioning suicide risk, indicated for patients with schizophrenia; also underutilized.

    c. Ketamine: Rapid reduction of depressive symptoms and suicidal ideation. Esketamine is FDA-approved with indications for adults with Treatment-Resistant Depression, and for depressive symptoms in adults with MDD with suicidal thoughts or actions.

    d. Antidepressants: Antidepressants can be used judiciously and effectively to address depression and anxiety, and on a population level, suicide preventive effects are associated with increased population rates of antidepressant use.

5. **Limit the quantity of medications dispensed during times of higher suicide risk**. Since suicide risk is dynamic, there may be periods of time during a patient's course when risk becomes more acute. During these periods it is important to stay more closely in communication with the patient and if possible, the patient's family, and limit the quantity of each medication refill, especially for medications with a narrow therapeutic index.

6. **Schedule meetings with the patient more frequently than usual**. When a medication is being initiated, when the dose is being increased, and when medications are being tapered down, these are periods when not only risk

of side effects is greater, but when underlying suicide risk can be perturbed by side effects such as anxiety, agitation or insomnia. Therefore these are important periods of time to see the patient more frequently, to communicate more closely, and to alert the patient when to contact you. Let the patient know how to reach you or the covering provider between visits.

7. During medication initiation or dosage changes, be sure to include the following in your communication with patients:

    a. Permission to speak with family or other support person if necessary.

    b. Consent to communicate with other health providers, e.g., therapist, primary care provider or psychiatrist.

    c. Education about transition periods during treatment, what to expect in the short-term and goals for the longer term.

    d. Encouragement and education about your goals for the treatment plan, ideas for next steps, offer the patient hope for improvement, remission, recovery.

8. Medication transitions are an excellent time to re-visit or initiate a patient's Safety Plan (see Chapter 7 for Safety Planning).

Note: recommendations related to medications included in this book are not comprehensive. Please see *Stahl Prescriber's Guide* for detailed prescribing guidance.[4]

C Lithium

A large body of evidence indicates that lithium decreases suicide in patients with affective disorders. Lithium has been suggested to have antisuicidal properties based on secondary analyses of RCTs, naturalistic studies, meta-analyses, and open-label treatment trials, likely related to and additionally independent of its mood-stabilizing effect.[5–11] Because lithium is generally used in patients with affective disorders, the antisuicidal effects of lithium have not been evaluated in patients with other psychiatric conditions such as schizophrenia.

Summary of the data related to lithium's impact on suicide:

1. Lithium is an effective mood stabilizer for bipolar disorder, and has effectiveness as an augmentation agent for unipolar depression. Stabilizing mood symptoms especially over the long term can contribute to suicide risk reduction.

2. Lithium has a large evidence base for having a protective effect against suicide drawn from more than 50 studies.[12,13]

3. Reduces suicide rates 60–80% in studies comparing lithium to placebo as well as lithium to other medications.[14]

4. Suicide attempt rates are also significantly reduced.

5. These suicide preventive effects are likely present for both unipolar and bipolar mood disorders.[15]

6. Lithium's suicide protective mechanism of action is not certain, but is possibly related to its effects in reducing aggression and impulsivity.

Lithium's Evidence for Suicide Risk Reduction

- In addition to stabilizing mood, lithium has a large evidence base for providing a protective effect against suicide among bipolar and unipolar depressed patients.

- While the majority of the studies are not RCTs and therefore have limitations, the risk-reducing effects are consistent and robust enough for expert opinion to support lithium as an effective intervention for suicide risk.

- Studies found reductions in both attempts and suicide deaths compared with placebo as well as compared with other older mood stabilizers.

● Clinical Considerations

Patients with mood disorders have as high as a 30 times greater risk of suicide[15] compared with the general population. Lithium is considered a first-line treatment option in several international guidelines,[16] and is a well-known augmentation strategy for unipolar depression. For any patient with a mood disorder and a history of past or current suicide risk, these significant potentially lifesaving benefits of lithium should be weighed against its side effect and medication risk profile.

Adverse effects especially with long-term use of lithium include possible renal and cardiac effects, and hyponatremia. Common side effects include nausea, tremor, thirst, weight gain, diarrhea, and dermatologic side effects. Additionally its relatively narrow therapeutic index along with these potential long-term effects require regular blood test monitoring of lithium levels and checks on renal and thyroid laboratory studies. Lithium toxicity can be dangerous and requires medical evaluation and treatment; early symptoms include diarrhea, nausea/vomiting, muscle weakness, drowsiness, incoordination, and muscle twitching. (See *Stahl Prescriber's Guide* for detailed guidance about prescribing lithium since there are potential long-term adverse effects that must be regularly monitored.)[4]

Its adverse effects, requirements for blood monitoring, narrow therapeutic index, relative lack of industry profit potential, and perhaps stigma related to lithium, have most likely been the reasons that lithium remains highly underutilized, especially given the strength of evidence for its robust suicide risk-reducing potential. Perhaps the fact that suicide prevention has not been a primary independent clinical target until recent years has also contributed to its underutilization.

Clinical Takeaways: Lithium and Suicide Prevention

- Consider lithium for targeting suicide risk reduction for patients with any mood disorder.
- Closely consider, assess, and monitor risk of suicide in any patient with a mood disorder, given the fact that half to two-thirds of all suicides occur in patients with mood disorders.
- Also consider lithium if full remission has not been achieved for a mood disorder patient, especially when suicide risk is present.
- Would generally consider the use of lithium for longer term improvements, not necessarily as a short-term antisuicidal agent. It is not clear how rapidly lithium works on suicide risk, given the methodological limitations of the data.
- Follow usual baseline laboratory and regular lithium monitoring including renal, thyroid, and other metabolic side effects.

 Clozapine

Clozapine was the first medication to receive a suicide preventive indication and from 2003 until 2020 it was the only medication in the USA with a suicide preventive indication, related to its risk-reducing potential in patients with schizophrenia. Clozapine is also known for its use in improving symptoms in treatment refractory patients with schizophrenia and schizoaffective disorder, as well as for its efficacy for negative symptoms. Schizophrenia and schizoaffective disorders are certainly among the more potent health condition risk factors for suicide with as many as 50% of people living with schizophrenia attempting suicide and approximately 10–13% dying by suicide.[17] Traditional (or first generation) antipsychotics such as haloperidol have not been shown to reduce suicide risk. When the atypical antipsychotic medications were noted to improve cognition in a way the older antipsychotic class had not, other effects were speculated and then observed. Early excitement about clozapine's potential to reduce suicide risk by as much as 80% in patients with schizophrenia was described by several groups including Meltzer et al.[18]

In a landmark study by Meltzer et al., 980 patients with schizophrenia or schizoaffective disorder were randomized to clozapine versus olanzapine. Of the nearly 1000 patients, 27% had been refractory to previous medications and were considered high risk for suicide based on prior attempts or current ideation. They were studied over a two-year period under matched study conditions. Results showed significantly fewer patients treated with clozapine attempted suicide (38% fewer, 34 versus 55 on olanzapine), and fewer required hospitalization or rescue interventions, antidepressants, or anxiolytics. Although five clozapine and three olanzapine subjects died by suicide during the two-year period, clozapine is still considered to have reduced risk overall, since those numbers were much smaller and lethality of method, possibly as, or more, important than intent, is known to have a large bearing on attempts being lethal versus surviving the attempt.[18]

Despite the strong evidence base leading to FDA regulatory approval for schizophrenia patients with a history of recurrent suicidal behavior clozapine has been an underutilized medication.[19] One impediment to the evidence-based use of clozapine for suicide risk and treatment-resistant schizophrenia has been clinician fear of serious adverse effects (e.g., severe neutropenia), and lack of knowledge about how to manage more common adverse effects such as sialorrhea, constipation, and tachycardia.[20] There has been a resurgence of interest in supporting clozapine prescribing, with initiatives in New York state and the Netherlands that provide call centers and education materials.[21–23]

Clinical Takeaways: Clozapine and Suicide Prevention

- Clozapine should be considered for any patient with schizophrenia or schizoaffective disorder, especially those patients who have known suicide risk.

- Keep in mind that schizophrenia and schizoaffective disorders are health conditions known to elevate suicide risk significantly, and therefore all patients with these chronic psychotic conditions should have their suicide risk assessed on an ongoing basis.

Please see *The Clozapine Handbook* (Meyer & Stahl) released in May 2019 that covers all aspects of clozapine prescribing in detail.[24] A new online resource has also emerged (https://smiadviser.org) supported by grants from the US Substance Abuse and Mental Health Services Administration (SAMHSA) and the American Psychiatric Association (APA). This online resource not only provides educational modules about clozapine, but also allows clinicians to register for free in order to obtain consultations about patients.

Ketamine

Ketamine induces rapid-onset and short-duration improvement in depressive and suicidal symptoms in Treatment-Resistant Depression and likely other mood disorders as well, and reduces chronic pain after short intravenous infusions.[25] In 2016, ketamine received a fast track designation by the FDA and in 2019 nasal esketamine (Spravato) was FDA-approved in the USA for Treatment-Resistant Depression in conjunction with other antidepressant medications. And in 2020 esketamine also received FDA approval with an indication for treating depressive symptoms in adults with MDD with suicidal thoughts or behaviors. Ketamine is now available in intravenous (ketamine) and intranasal (esketamine) forms.

● **History of Ketamine**

Ketamine has a colorful history originally launched as an anesthetic in 1970, with not only analgesic and sedation effects, but bronchodilation, anti-inflammatory, and later found to have neuroprotective effects. Used on soldiers in Vietnam, and adult and pediatric surgical and burn cases, general, spinal, and regional anesthetic indications, then in veterinary medicine use in animals, it soon became a recreational club drug related to its hallucinogenic properties. A "dissociative" anesthetic, people may disconnect from their environment leading to usually transient dissociative symptoms. In recent years, ketamine has shown significant therapeutic effects in major depression, bipolar disorder, anxiety, and PTSD.

Ketamine has clear therapeutic benefits for depression with response rates from 50–70% within hours to single dose even in patients who have not responded to more than one prior antidepressant.[26–28] However, antidepressant effects last only a few days.

There is both excitement in the clinical field and the public related to its potential to improve Treatment-Resistant Depression and depression with suicidal ideation, and concern related to side effects especially over the long term, the short-term nature of the response, and practical accessibility given the mode of delivery is limited to intravenous and intranasal only available under physician supervision at approved health centers.[29,30] Additionally, concern arose related to the rise in clinical providers starting around 2010, some of whom are not trained in mental health.[31] A 2017 consensus statement examined the data and limitations related to ketamine's use in mood disorders and expresses a cautious approach due to concerns about small sample sizes, shortage of long-term data and substance abuse potential.[32]

● Mechanism of Action

NMDA receptor antagonist and glutamate modulator. NMDA receptors are present at high densities in the PFC, pyramidal cells, and hippocampus, and blocking NMDA in these areas could theoretically lead to increases in GLU output. Theoretically it may have antidepressant effects at low (subanesthetic) doses related to glutamate activity. However not all NMDA receptors have demonstrated a clear antidepressant effect. Potential other mechanisms include binding at many different receptor sites: mu opioid, 5HT, NE, alpha-7, nicotinic, muscarinic receptors – a typical "dirty drug" in the MOA sense.

At different doses it potentially has different effects from nocioceptive, to anesthetic, to hallucinogenic.

● Intravenous Ketamine Dosing for Treatment Refractory Depression

Krystal et al. initially settled on what became the recommended dosing strategy of 0.5 mg/kg ketamine infused intravenously over 40 minutes, derived from earlier psychosis studies, aiming for therapeutic benefits without producing delirium or an anesthetized state.[33] Frequency of dosing for early phase initiation of treatment ranges from one–three times/week and maintenance dosing frequency ranges from weekly to once every six weeks.[32]

● Side Effects of Ketamine and Esketamine

- increased blood pressure, increased cardiac output
- increased intracranial pressure
- tachycardia or bradycardia
- N/V (no p.o. intake 30 min pre- and 2 hrs post-)
- cognitive problems, perceptual effects, hallucinations
- sedation
- vivid dreams
- i.v. ketamine only: respiratory depression or apnea with large doses or rapid infusion

Long-term safety is not well known. Also relatively unknown is ketamine's impact on suicidal behavior, as it is mainly known to improve suicidal ideation.

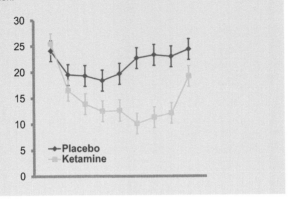

Figure 9.2 Rapid antidepressant effect for unmedicated treatment resistant patients with MDD

Zarate et al. found a rapid change in depressive symptoms following intravenous ketamine infusion.[26]

● Esketamine

Esketamine is FDA-approved for adjunctive treatment of TRD as well as for depressive symptoms in adults with MDD with suicidal thoughts or behaviors, and is delivered intranasally under the supervision of an approved clinical provider. It is not obtained from a regular outpatient pharmacy for at home use. It is administered in a health clinic setting; length of visit is 2–2.5 hours. In addition to showing benefit for adjunctive treatment of TRD, for patients with TRD who experienced remission or response after esketamine treatment, continuation of esketamine nasal spray in addition to oral antidepressant treatment delayed relapse compared with antidepressant plus placebo.[34] Induction dosing is recommended twice/week for four weeks, and maintenance dosing is once/week or once every two weeks. Flexible dosing is available after the starting dose of 56 mg.

For details of esketamine's safety and efficacy data, dosing, and administration, please go to the FDA site www.fda.gov/media/121379/download and to find a health center that provides esketamine, go to www.spravatohcp.com.

Figure 9.3 Effect of ketamine on suicidal ideation

Effect of ketamine on suicidal thoughts

Wilkinson reviewed multiple studies and found these rapid, positive effects on suicidal ideation.[31]

Effect of a single dose of ketamine on suicidal ideation, as indicated by clinician-administered measure[a]

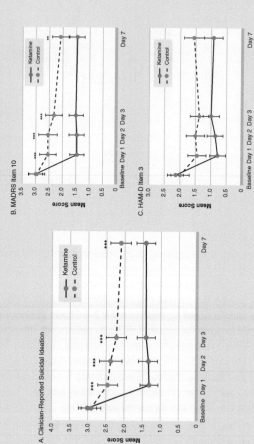

Antidepressants

Antidepressants as a class have beneficial effects for the treatment of depression, and some are effective for panic disorder, generalized anxiety, social phobia, obsessive compulsive disorder (OCD), PTSD, premenstrual dysphoric disorder, vasomotor symptoms, and binge eating disorder.[35] Concerns about degree of efficacy especially for milder forms of depression have been countered by analyses that find increasing placebo response rates led to smaller effect size.[36,37] A 2018 systematic review and meta-analysis of 522 published and unpublished double-blind RCTs found all antidepressants were more effective than placebo, with overall OR of 1.66 for response and 1.56 for remission.[1] One estimate is that antidepressants alone or with augmentation benefit 60–70% of patients with MDD.[38]

All medications have various side effects and individual variability exists, but a thorough umbrella review of 45 meta-analyses spanning over 1000 studies of antidepressant safety confirmed the overall safety of antidepressants.[39] While this does not mean antidepressants do not have side effects which can be significant nor that some individuals may have more serious side effects, it does mean that the concerns related to several possible adverse health outcomes including the concern about suicide risk were found to not be supported by convincing evidence.

● Evidence for Antidepressants' Reduction of Suicide Risk

In an ecologic study comparing suicide rates against antidepressant prescription rates at the county level in the USA, investigators found higher antidepressant prescription rates were correlated with lower suicide rates among all age demographics including among children.[40] Additionally a review of other correlative pharmacoepidemiological studies that compared suicide rates by region and year with the concurrent rates of prescriptions for antidepressants also found an inverse relationship between suicide rates and population antidepressant use.[41]

In a population-based study in Sweden, a researcher hypothesized that if antidepressant prescription use increased several fold, it could lead to a reduction in the national rate of suicide (by 25%). In a naturalistic course of events, rates of antidepressant use did increase 3.5-fold over a nearly 20 year period from 1978 to 1996, and the national rate did decrease by 19%. While other strategies may have also come to bear, the increased use of antidepressants was considered to at least partially contribute to reduced suicides.[42] Another US population-based study of suicide risk during the initial phase of antidepressant treatment for 65,103 patients (adults and children) did not show an elevated risk of suicide or suicide attempts.[43]

● Antidepressants in Youth

Pharmacoepidemiological data from the USA suggest that paralleling the widespread use of SSRIs, suicide rates among those aged 15–19 years fell from 11/100,000 in 1990 to 7.3/100,000 in 2003. Synchronous with the US FDA black box warning on antidepressants in 2004 and the reduction in antidepressant usage, suicide rates increased.[44] A meta-analysis found the use of fluoxetine to treat pediatric patients with MDD neither increased nor significantly decreased the risk of suicidal behavior.[45]

Use of Antidepressants in Youth

Summary findings and recommendations by Dr. David Brent, a leading expert in pediatric suicide prevention:[45]

- Newer antidepressants are associated with a slightly increased risk of suicidal events (but not suicide) compared with placebo in RCTs in youth.
- Four to eleven times more depressed youth benefit from antidepressants than experience a suicidal event.
- Pharmacoepidemiologic studies, which are much larger and more representative of patient populations than RCTs, show a protective effect of regional antidepressant use on suicide.
- Youth most likely to experience a suicidal event in the early phase of medical treatment have high baseline suicidal ideation, family conflict, alcohol and substance use, nonsuicidal self-injury, and non-response to treatment.
- Clinicians can mitigate suicide risk in depressed youths through education, safety planning, close clinical monitoring, targeting of suicidal risk factors, and rational dosing.

For full prescribing information for medications in child and adolescent populations, please see *Prescriber's Guide – Children and Adolescents: Stahl's Essential Pharmacology.*[46]

Key Point

Consensus among many experts is that several methods such as ecological studies and long-term very large database studies provide evidence that antidepressants reduce suicide risk overall.[47,48]

G Antidepressants and Warnings: US Food & Drug Administration (FDA) "Black Box" and UK Medicines and Healthcare Products Regulatory Authority (MHRA) Warnings on Antidepressant Medications Related to Suicide Risk in Youth

In 2003 and 2004 federal regulatory agencies in Europe and the USA issued a series of warnings about the use of antidepressant medications in young people related to suicide risk ultimately leading to the US black box warning in 2004. In 2006, the FDA expanded the warning to include 36 antidepressants and raised the age of potentially vulnerable patients from 18 to 24.[49] These decisions were based on data from RCTs by the drug makers, which found increased incidence of suicidal ideation and behavior in subjects on newer antidepressants compared with placebo. However, the decisions were controversial because the methodology of these clinical trials did not include the ability to measure improvements in suicidal states, only the emergence of adverse events. And other studies have found beneficial effects related both to depressive, anxiety, and eating disorders – all conditions that are potent risk factors for suicide. Further, population level pharmacoepidemiologic studies have found regional associations between higher rates of antidepressant prescribing and **decreased** rates of suicide.[50,51] Advocacy organizations raised concerns that the progress that had been made especially in primary care with more aggressive identification and treatment of depression as one of the world's leading causes of disability and a major driver of suicide risk, might be hindered. And in fact, a substantial drop in diagnosing depression and use of antidepressants (and other non-pharmacological treatments for depression) followed the warnings, and instead of declining as hoped, suicide attempts and suicides have increased.[52–54]

● Unintended Effects of Antidepressant Warnings

A number of studies in the years that followed the warnings examined issues such as rates of diagnosis, treatment, and prescribing, as well as patient outcomes. A very large cohort study of 7.5 million patients in the US by Lu et al. found both prescribing of antidepressants and diagnosing depression declined. In the second year after the FDA black box warnings were issued, prescription rates of antidepressants **decreased** from baseline rates by 31% in adolescents aged 10–17 and by 24.3% in young adults aged 18–29. Prescription rates also decreased by 14.5% in adults aged 30–64 even though the warning did not refer to them. Therefore a spillover effect into older age groups seemed to occur.[52]

Other studies did not find a compensatory increase in the use of other treatments for depression such as psychotherapy, ECT, or other medications, and data from those studies also suggest that doctors became less likely to diagnose and treat their patients for depression.[53]

While causality is not examined as this is only by temporal association and suicidal behavior has multiple underpinnings, suicide attempts among people aged 10 to 29 in this very large patient cohort rose – by 22% in adolescents, and by 34% in young adults. Suicide attempts using other methods and attempts that did not result in a visit to the healthcare systems were not included, so the actual rates were most likely higher. There was no significant change in the rate of suicide in the study.[52]

Another study looking at both European and US warnings found SSRI prescriptions for youths decreased by approximately 22% in both the USA and the Netherlands, and by 51% in the UK after the warnings were issued.[55] In the Netherlands, the youth suicide rate increased by 49% between 2003 and 2005 and showed a significant inverse association with SSRI prescriptions. In the USA, after a decrease in youth suicide rates by 28% from 1990 to 2003, youth suicide rates increased by 14% between 2003 and 2004.[50]

Clinical Takeaways

1. Screen for and aggressively manage depression.
2. Weigh the risk and benefits of all treatment options, non-pharmacological and medications, alongside the risks and benefits of the illness itself and also of not using a particular treatment.
3. Use antidepressant medications judiciously, starting with low doses and monitor closely especially in the first several weeks and with any dosage changes for side effects such as agitation, anxiety, or insomnia.
4. Monitor patients, especially youth and young adult patients, closely for suicidal ideation.
5. Provide education and support to patients (and families when possible) so that patients are monitoring for early changes and are able to communicate them with the clinical provider/team.

Role of the Media

During the 12–18-month period preceding the FDA black box warning, there was considerable media coverage while public hearings occurred at the FDA. Despite urging from the American Foundation for Suicide Prevention (AFSP) and other mental health and patient advocacy organizations to include both the risks and benefits of antidepressants in their considerations, the FDA issued a black box warning, its strongest possible warning, affixed to the packaging of antidepressants in 2004 in an effort to alert doctors and patients about the increased risk of suicidal thoughts. The media's coverage of the sensationalized controversy surrounding the decision-making process and the warning itself most likely impacted public perceptions and exaggerated concerns about antidepressants that have likely persisted over the years.

● FDA Black Box Warning

The data that led to the FDA's decision were a set of randomized clinical trials of antidepressants involving nearly 100,000 participants, which showed that the rate of suicidal thinking or suicidal behavior was 4% among patients assigned to receive an antidepressant, as compared with 2% among those assigned to receive placebo; there were notably no suicide deaths.[56] Subsequent age-stratified analyses showed that this increased risk was significant only among children and adolescents under the age of 18 years; there was no evidence of increased risk among adults older than 24 years, and in this FDA data set, among adults 65 years of age or older, antidepressants had a clear protective effect against the development of suicidal ideation and behavior.

Unintentionally, the FDA warnings and media coverage created a climate of fear about antidepressants, and exaggerated the risk of taking antidepressants among people suffering with depression, their health professionals, and the general public. Due to this impact among providers and families, opportunities to identify and treat depression were foregone, and this burden of unaddressed depression could have impacted the risk for suicidal behavior and suicides. This negative outcome was not exclusive to youth and young adults, since a spillover effect occurred which also decreased the rate of diagnosis and treatment of depression in middle aged adults.

Key Point: Educating and Monitoring Patients on Antidepressants

A more accurate interpretation of the studies presented to the FDA in 2003 might have led to a recommendation for close follow-up and education for patients and family members when starting a new medication. Careful monitoring for any emergence or worsening of suicidal thinking and symptoms such as agitation, anxiety, or insomnia is essential when prescribing antidepressants (and any psychotropic or other medication for that matter). This approach fosters communication and should always be the standard of care when any new medication is started.

This is a cautionary tale of unintended consequences that occurred when controversial interpretation of data led to regulatory warnings, inflamed by media reporting that grossly sensationalized the warning and simplified the data, ultimately impacting physician behavior and the public attitude toward the treatment of one of the most disabling medical conditions worldwide, depression. Some experts have argued that since the 2007 revision of the FDA warning, adding the consideration that depression itself has its own risk of suicide, does not seem to have had the impact of improvement in consideration of the balance between the serious risk of unaddressed depression and the relatively small risk associated with antidepressant treatment, that the FDA should consider removing the black box warning altogether.[57,58]

KEY TAKEAWAYS

a. Depression and many other psychiatric conditions can be fatal.

b. Treating these health conditions as well as focusing on the clinical target of suicide risk more specifically and separately, can save lives.

c. Several medications have clear data that point to suicide risk reduction, and yet some of these, lithium and clozapine notably, remain underutilized.

d. Many studies over several decades offer a body of information and demonstrate that treatment with antidepressants can help effectively manage depression and reduces the risk of suicide.

e. Unfortunately, confusion still lingers related to antidepressants and suicide risk that have had consequences of decreased rates of diagnosing and treating depression, even beyond the age limit (24 and under) of the FDA's warning.

f. When the FDA was considering the decision about whether to issue the black box warnings, the studies used in making the decision only examined the adverse events associated with medication, but failed to take into account the positive impact of treatment.

g. Several new medications focused on mood and suicide risk, such as ketamine, offer hope for the development of more pharmacological treatments that will reduce suicide risk in high risk patients.

References

Overarching Guidelines for Medications and Suicide Prevention

1   Li, G., Fife, D., Wang, G., et al. (2019) All-cause mortality in patients with treatment-resistant depression: a cohort study in the US population. *Annals of General Psychiatry*, 18: 23. doi: 10.1186/s12991-019-0248-0

2   Kellner, C. H., Fink, M., Knapp, R., et al. (2005) Relief of expressed suicidal intent by ECT: a consortium for research in ECT study. *Am J Psychiatry*, 162(5): 977–82. doi: 10.1176/appi.ajp.162.5.977

3   George, M. S., Raman, R., Benedek, D. M., et al. (2014) A two-site pilot randomized 3 day trial of high dose left prefrontal repetitive transcranial magnetic stimulation (rTMS) for suicidal inpatients. *Brain Stimul*, 7(3): 421–31.

4   Stahl, S. M. (2017) *Stahl's Essential Psychopharmacology Prescriber's Guide*, 6th Edn. Cambridge, UK: Cambridge University Press.

Lithium

5   Thies-Flechtner, K., Müller-Oerlinghausen, B., Seibert, W., Walther, A., & Greil, W. (1996) Effect of prophylactic treatment on suicide risk in patients with major affective disorders: data from a randomized prospective trial. *Pharmacopsychiatry*, 29: 103–7.

6   Müller-Oerlinghausen, B., Muser-Causemann, B., & Volk, J. (1992) Suicides and parasuicides in a high-risk patient group on and off lithium long-term medication. *J Affect Disord*, 25: 261–69.

7   Goodwin, F. K., Fireman, B., Simon, G. E., Hunkeler, E. M., Lee, J., & Revicki, D. (2003) Suicide risk in bipolar disorder during treatment with lithium and divalproex. *JAMA*, 290: 1467–73.

8   Baldessarini, R. J., Tondo, L., Faedda, G. L., Suppes, T. R., Floris, G., & Rudas, N. (1996) Effects of the rate of discontinuing lithium maintenance treatment in bipolar disorders. *J Clin Psychiatry*, 57: 441–48.

9   Cipriani, A., Pretty, H., Hawton, K., & Geddes, J. R. (2005) Lithium in the prevention of suicidal behavior and all-cause mortality in patients with mood disorders: a systematic review of randomized trials. *Am J Psychiatry*, 162: 1805–19.

10 Baldessarini, R. J., Tondo, L., Davis, P., Pompili, M., Goodwin, F. K., & Hennen, J. (2006) Decreased risk of suicides and attempts during long-term lithium treatment: a meta-analytic review. *Bipolar Disord*, 8: 625–39.

11 Cipriani, A., Hawton, K., Stockton, S., & Geddes, J. R. (2013) Lithium in the prevention of suicide in mood disorders: Updated systematic review and meta-analysis. *BMJ*, 346: f3646.

12 Lewitzka, U., Severus, E., Bauer, R., Ritter, P., Müller-Oerlinghausen, B., & Bauer, M. (2015) The suicide prevention effect of lithium: more than 20 years of evidence–a narrative review. *International Journal of Bipolar Disorders*, 3(1): 32. doi: 10.1186/s40345-015-0032-2

13 Baldessarini, R. J., Tondo, L., Davis, P., Pompili, M., Goodwin, F. K., & Hennen, J. (2006) Decreased risk of suicides and attempts during long-term lithium treatment: a meta-analytic review. *Bipolar Disord*, 8(5 Pt 2): 625–39.

14 Guzzetta, F., Tondo, L., Centorrino, F., & Baldessarini, R. J. (2007) Lithium treatment reduces suicide risk in recurrent major depressive disorder. *J Clin Psychiatry*, 68(3): 380–83.

15 Isometsä, E. (2014) Suicidal behaviour in mood disorders: Who, when, and why? *Canadian Journal of Psychiatry. Revue canadienne de psychiatrie*, 59(3): 120–30. doi.org/10.1177/070674371405900303

16   Lam, R. W., Kennedy, S. H., Grigoriadis, S., et al. (2009) Canadian Network for Mood and Anxiety Treatments (CANMAT) clinical guidelines for the management of major depressive disorder in adults. III: pharmacopsychiatry. *J Affect Disord*, 117: 26–43. doi: 10.1016/j.jad.2009.06.041

Clozapine

17   Pompili, M., Amador, X. F., Girardi, P., et al. (2007) Suicide risk in schizophrenia: learning from the past to change the future. *Annals of General Psychiatry*, 6: 10. doi: 10.1186/1744-859X-6-10

18   Meltzer, H. Y., & Okayli, G. (1995) Reduction of suicidality during clozapine treatment of neuroleptic-resistant schizophrenia: impact on risk-benefit assessment. *Am J Psychiatry* 152(2): 183–90.

19   Correll, C. U., & Kane, J. M. (2019) Ranking antipsychotics for efficacy and safety in schizophrenia. *JAMA Psychiatry*. Published online November 06, 2019, doi.org/10.1001/jamapsychiatry.2019.3377

20   Leung, J. G., Cusimano, J., Gannon, J. M., et al. (2019) Addressing clozapine under-prescribing and barriers to initiation: a psychiatrist, advanced practice provider, and trainee survey. *Int Clin Psychopharmacol*, 34: 247–56.

21   Gee, S., Vergunst, F., Howes, O., & Taylor, D. (2014) Practitioner attitudes to clozapine initiation. *Acta Psychiatr Scand*, 130: 16–24.

22   Cohen, D. (2014) Prescribers fear as a major side-effect of clozapine. *Acta Psychiatr Scand*, 130: 154–55.

23   Carruthers, J., Radigan, M., Erlich, M. D., et al. (2016) An initiative to improve clozapine prescribing in New York State. *Psychiatr Serv*, 67: 369–71.

24   Meyer, J. M., & Stahl, S. M. (2019) *The Clozapine Handbook*. New York, NY; Cambridge University Press.

Ketamine/Esketamine

25   Stahl, S. (2013) Mechanism of action of ketamine. *CNS Spectrums*, 18(4): 171–74. doi: 10.1017/S109285291300045X

26   Zarate, C. A., Singh, J. B., Carlson, P. J., et al. (2006) A randomized trial of an N-methyl-D-aspartate antagonist in treatment-resistant major depression. *Arch Gen Psychiatry*, 63(8): 856–64.

27   Ionescu, D. F., Luckenbaugh, D. A., Niciu, M. J., Richards, E. M., & Zarate, C. A., Jr (2015) A single infusion of ketamine improves depression scores in patients with anxious bipolar depression. *Bipolar Disorders*, 17(4): 438–43. doi: 10.1111/bdi.12277

28   Murrough, J. W., Iosifescu, D. V., Chang, L. C., et al. (2013) Antidepressant efficacy of ketamine in treatment-resistant major depression: a two-site randomized controlled trial. *Am J Psychiatry*, 170(10): 1134–42. doi: 10.1176/appi.ajp.2013.13030392

29   Ballard, E. D., Yarrington, J. S., Farmer, C. A., et al. (2018) Characterizing the course of suicidal ideation response to ketamine. *J Affect Disord*, 241: 86–93. doi: 10.1016/j.jad.2018.07.077. Epub 2018 Jul 30.

30   Ballard, E. D., Ionescu, D. F., Vande Voort, J. L., et al. (2014) Improvement in suicidal ideation after ketamine infusion: Relationship to reductions in depression and anxiety. *J Psychiatr Res*, 58: 161–66. doi: 10.1016/j.jpsychires.2014.07.027. Epub Aug 12, 2014.

31   Wilkinson, S. T., Toprak, M., Turner, M. S., Levine, S. P., Katz, R. B., & Sanacora, G. (2017) A survey of the clinical, off-label use of ketamine as a treatment for psychiatric disorders. *Am J Psychiatry*, 174(7): 695–96. doi: 10.1176/appi.ajp.2017.17020239

32   Sanacora, G., Frye, M. A., McDonald, W., Mathew, S. J., Turner, M. S., & Schatzberg, A. F., (2017) A consensus statement on the use of ketamine in the treatment of mood disorders. *American Psychiatric Association Council of Research Task Force on Novel Biomarkers and Treatments. JAMA Psychiatry*, 74(4): 399–405. doi: 10.1001/jamapsychiatry.2017.0080

33   Krystal, J. H., Abdallah, C. G., Sanacora, G., Charney, D. S., & Duman, R. S. (2019) Ketamine: A paradigm shift for depression research and treatment. *Neuroview*, 101(5): 774–78.

34   Daly, E. J., Trivedi, M. H., Janik, A., et al. (2019) Efficacy of esketamine nasal spray plus oral antidepressant treatment for relapse prevention in patients with treatment-resistant depression: a randomized clinical trial. *JAMA Psychiatry*, 76(9): 893–903. Advance online publication. doi: 10.1001/jamapsychiatry.2019.1189

Antidepressants

35   Cipriani, A., Furukawa, T. A., Salanti, G., et al. (2018) Comparative efficacy and acceptability of 21 antidepressant drugs for the acute treatment of adults with major depressive disorder: A systematic review and network meta-analysis. *Lancet*, 391(10128): 1357–66.

36   Davey, C. G., & Chanen, A. M. (2016) The unfulfilled promise of the antidepressant medications. *Med J*, 204: 348–50.

37   Wang, S. M., Han, C., Lee, S. J., et al. (2018) Efficacy of antidepressants: bias in randomized clinical trials and related issues. *Expert Rev Clin Pharmacol*, 11: 15–25.

38   Ionescu, D. F., & Papakostas, G. L. (2017) Experimental medication treatment approaches for depression. *Transl Psychiatry*, 7: e1068.

39   Dragioti, E., Solmi, M., Favaro, A., et al. (2019) Association of antidepressant use with adverse health outcomes: a systematic umbrella review. *JAMA Psychiatry*. Published online October 02, 2019. doi: 10.1001/jamapsychiatry.2019.2859

40   Gibbons, R. D., Hur, K., Bhaumik, D. K., & Mann, J. J. (2006) The relationship between antidepressant prescription rates and rate of early adolescent suicide. *Am J Psychiatry*, 163(11): 1898–904.

41   Baldessarini, R. J., & Tondo, L. (2007). Psychopharmacology of suicide prevention. In R. Tatarelli, M. Pompili & P. Girardi (Eds.), *Suicide in Psychiatric Disorder* New York: Nova Science Publications, 193–213.

42   Isacsson, G. (2000) Suicide prevention: A medical breakthrough? *Acta Psychiatrica Scandinavica*, 102: 113–17. doi: 10.1034/j.1600-0447.2000.102002113.x

43   Simon, G. E., Savarino, J., Operskalski, B., & Wang, P. S. (2006) Suicide risk during antidepressant treatment. *Am J Psychiatry*, 163(1): 41–7.

44   Hamilton, B. E., Miniño, A. M., Martin, J. A., Kochanek, K. D., Strobino, D. M., & Guyer, B. (2007) Annual summary of vital statistics: 2005. *Pediatrics*, 119 (2): 345–60. doi: 10.1542/peds.2006-3226

45   Brent, D. A. (2016) Antidepressants and suicidality. *Psychiatric Clinics*, 39(3): 503–12.

46   Stahl, S. M. (2018) *Prescriber's Guide – Children and Adolescents: Stahl's Essential Psychopharmacology*. Cambridge, UK: Cambridge University Press.

47   Isacsson, G., & Rich, C. L. (2005) Antidepressant drug use and suicide prevention. *International Review of Psychiatry*, 17(3): 153–62. doi: 10.1080/09540260500071608

48   Olin, B., Jayewardene, A. K., Bunker, M., & Moreno, F. (2012) Mortality and suicide risk in treatment-resistant depression: an observational study of the long-term impact of intervention. *PLoS one*, 7(10): e48002. doi: 10.1371/journal.pone.0048002

Antidepressants and US/UK Warnings

49 Food and Drug Administration. (2016) Revisions to product labeling. Retrieved from www.fda .gov/downloads/Drugs/DrugSafety/InformationbyDrugClass/UCM173233.pdf.

50 Gibbons, R. D., Hur, K., Bhaumik, D. K., & Mann, J. J. (2016) The relationship between antidepressant prescription rates and rate of early adolescent suicide. *Am J Psychiatry*, 163(11): 1898–904.

51 Ludwig, J., Marcotte, D. E., & Norberg, K. (2009) Anti-depressants and suicide. *J Health Econ*, 28(3): 659–76.

52 Lu, C. Y., Zhang, F., Lakoma, M. D., Madden, J. M., Rusinak, D., Penfold, R. B., et al. (2014) Changes in antidepressant use by young people and suicidal behavior after FDA warnings and media coverage: Quasi-experimental study. *BMJ*, 348: g3596. doi: 10.1136/bmj.g3596

53 Valuck, R. J., Libby, A. M., Sills, M. R., Giese, A. A., & Allen, R. R. (2004) Antidepressant treatment and risk of suicide attempt by adolescents with major depressive disorder. *CNS Drugs*, 18: 1119–32. doi: 10.2165/00023210–200418150-00006

54 Gibbons, R. D., Brown, C. H., Hur, K., Marcus, S. M., Bhaumik, D. K., & Mann, J. J. (2007) Relationship between antidepressants and suicide attempts: An analysis of the Veterans Health Administration data sets. *Am J Psychiatry*, 164(7): 1044–49. doi: 10.1176/ajp.2007.164.7.1044

55 Bergen, H., Hawton, K., Murphy, E., et al. (2009) Trends in prescribing and self-poisoning in relation to UK regulatory authority warnings against use of SSRI antidepressants in under-18-year-olds. *Br J Clin Pharmacol*, 68(4): 618–29. doi: 10.1111/j.1365-2125.2009.03481.x

56 Hammad, T. A. (2004) Review and evaluation of clinical data [Internet]. Silver Spring: US Food and Drug Administration. Available from: www.fda.gov/ohrms/dockets/ac/04/briefing/2004-4065b1-10-TAB08-Hammads-Review.pdf.

57 Friedman, R. A. (2014) Antidepressants' black-box warning: 10 years later. *N Engl J Med*, 371: 1666–68.

58 Valuck, R. J., Libby, A. M., Orton, H. D., Morrato, E. H., Allen, R., & Baldessarini, R. J. (2007) Spillover effects on treatment of adult depression in primary care after FDA advisory on risk of pediatric suicidality with SSRIs. *Am J Psychiatry*, 164: 1198–205.

10

Suicide Prevention in Healthcare Systems

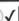

 ## Introduction

● **A Health Systems Approach: Widening the Lens on Suicide Prevention**

Perspectives on suicide prevention in health and behavioral health systems have widened in recent years from focusing primarily on the skills and practices of individual providers to now taking in the goal of creating a suicide-safer healthcare system as a whole. This movement has been inspired by other quality initiatives in healthcare that aim to eliminate medical errors, improve continuity, and improve organizational innovation by reducing the occurrence of preventable untoward outcomes. In the field of suicide prevention, this movement has included the aspirational goal of "zero suicides" in care.

 ## PRINCIPLES

- Suicide prevention frameworks are increasingly focusing on creating safer systems of care, which involves developing a culture of safety and prevention, implementing effective policies and practices, and building up a workforce that is continually engaged and supported with education and development.

- A systems approach to suicide prevention is rooted in patient safety "zero defect care" principles that encourage a commitment to the aspirational goal of "zero suicides."

Figure 10.1. Suicide prevention in health systems (zero suicide)

Suicide prevention in health systems involves commitment to a culture of safety and prevention; best practice, pathways, and policies; and workforce engagement and education. Lived experience and continuous improvement play an important role in each of these areas.

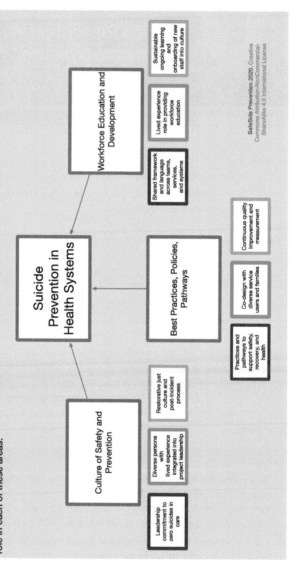

- The integration of lived experience of suicide into leadership teams, care system design, and workforce education is critical if prevention efforts are to match the needs of patients.

- A constructive, responsive, and non-blaming process for responding to suicide events is essential for systems aiming toward a zero suicide goal.

- While treatment pathways defined by risk stratification can provide useful starting points, resources should be allocated based on assessments of individual circumstances.

- Services should be designed not just with the needs of at-risk persons in mind, but by working **with** service users, family members, and others with lived experience related to suicide.

- Reaching toward the goal of zero suicides in care requires a continuous quality improvement mindset and commitment.

- Effective care at the systems level requires a shared language and conceptual framework that enables all parts of the systems to communicate effectively and work toward the same ends.

- Workforce education should include education by those with a lived experience of suicide risk.

- "One and done" training should be replaced with educational models that promote continuous learning and the onboarding of new staff into a shared culture of prevention.

C Culture of Safety and Prevention

A health systems approach to suicide prevention calls for the transformation of health, behavioral health, and community organizations so that prevention is considered a core responsibility and priority. This involves making a sustained organizational commitment to a culture of safety and the prevention of suicide. It also means pursuing a systems approach to care, with services being designed specifically to take account of the needs of individuals at risk for suicide, and ensuring that the structures available for the care of patients are appropriate to their needs.[1]

● Leadership Commitment

A commitment to work toward the prevention of all suicides (often called a "zero suicide" goal) does not assume that every suicide that has taken place in the past could have been prevented. Rather, it reflects a culture dedicated to quality improvement and patient safety. In order to foster such a culture, leaders at high levels should insist on: 1) the integration of lived experience perspectives into the system of care; 2) the development of processes directed at the goal of continuous quality improvement; and 3) the creation of a culture of supportive and restorative post-incident learning.

Toward Zero Suicides in Care in New South Wales, Australia

The government of New South Wales (NSW) in Australia invested AU$90 million in a set of coordinated initiatives aimed at moving toward the goal of zero suicides in the NSW health systems. These programs include a strong focus on workforce education in a common recovery-oriented framework (co-taught by persons with clinical and lived experience) and codesign of systems with those with lived experience of suicide. Initiatives include proactive follow-up and outreach measures and community-based care options such as alternatives to emergency department care. This whole system approach engages consumers and family members in every project and promotes a non-blaming, continuous learning approach to quality improvement and response to adverse events.

https://suicidepreventioncentralcoast.org.au/wp-content/uploads/2019/07/towards-zero.pdf

● From Zero Defect to Zero Suicide to Suicide Prevention in Health Systems

The goal of zero suicide has its roots in the wider "zero defect" approach to patient safety. Zero defect was originally developed as a quality control principle for aerospace and automobile manufacturing in the 1960s. The goal of achieving perfect outcomes in patient safety attracted interest in medical circles in the late 1990s and was first applied in a behavioral health context by the Henry Ford Health System in Detroit. Treating the death of a patient through suicide as the ultimate defective outcome of mental healthcare, clinicians in the system worked to implement what they called "Perfect Depression Care." The outcome of this program was a radical reduction in suicide deaths (80% over 10 years), and clinical studies soon provided supporting evidence for the effectiveness of the approach. In the years since, zero suicide has become an aspirational goal at both national and international levels.

AFSP Project 2025: Leadership and Collaboration Across Systems to Achieve Specific Goals

The ultimate goal of zero suicide can only be approached via incremental steps involving achievable targets that can be hit within an easily conceptualized horizon. A model project of this sort is the AFSP Project 2025, which aims to reduce suicide across the USA by 20% by 2025. Taking their start-point from the goals of the National Strategy for Suicide Prevention, the AFSP project seeks to provide an actionable plan for implementing this strategy. After extensive background research and the running of many simulations, AFSP identified four broad areas that had the potential for the greatest impact on suicide deaths: firearms, healthcare systems, emergency departments, and the corrections system. By working with strategic partners in each of these areas, the goal of the project is to bring about systemic changes. AFSP predicts that over 9,000 lives can be saved by taking two measures: 1) improving assessment and screening to a level that successfully identifies even one in five of the people at risk of suicide in large healthcare systems; and 2) providing those identified as at risk with brief interventions and improved follow-up care. The effectiveness of the approach identified by AFSP relies on the integration of training, implementation of new procedures, and care that is fundamentally connected at different stages and across different locations within each healthcare system.

10

● Objections and Alternatives to the Language of "Zero Suicide"

There are two common objections to the term "zero suicide" when it is first introduced to a health system. First, some argue that it is an unobtainable goal and that an excessive focus on an ideal distracts from realistic objectives. Second, clinicians and community members often worry that a zero suicide approach will entail consequences or blame if suicides do occur, as if it implies a "zero tolerance" policy.

These concerns are understandable. Achievable goals are vital and there has been an unfortunate history of clinicians being blamed in the aftermath of suicide. Nevertheless, there is no necessary conflict between an aspirational long-term goal and the supportive steps one might take to come closer to it right now. The direction of travel for short- and medium-term goals is clearly toward rather than away from zero suicides. When one target has been achieved, the next will surely be a step closer to zero. Dr. Kathy Turner, a leader in zero suicide system transformation at Gold Coast Mental Health (Australia), puts it this way: "When people object to the goal of zero suicide, my question for them is, what other goal would we have?"

Despite the importance of the goal, many health systems and localities opt not to use the language of "zero suicide" because of concerns about how that term will be understood and received by clinicians, patients, and community members. Decisions concerning how to brand a particular health systems approach must be made by local stakeholders with knowledge of the context and culture. For example, the New Zealand national strategy for suicide prevention, which was developed with a great deal of cultural stakeholder input, envisions "a future without suicide" under the broad heading "Every Life Matters." What is most important is that the strategy encompasses the key areas of a systems approach and that a system and/or region has an inclusive program that all stakeholders can rally around.

A Future Without Suicide

The decision to use the term "zero suicide" must be considered in a cultural context. The New Zealand national suicide prevention strategy envisions a "future without suicide," without reference to the term "zero suicide."

- A future without suicide
- Achieving a future where there is no suicide is an ambitious, long-term vision. When this vision is achieved, the suicide rate will have reduced, and every person and their whānau or family is more likely to have increased confidence and feel their life matters through:

  - **whakapapa** – having a strong identity, knowing where they come from and where they belong
  - **tūmanako** – having self-worth and being optimistic about their future
  - **whanaungatanga** – being connected with others: friends, whānau and families, and wider communities
  - **atawhaitanga** – receiving support that responds to their distress with compassion, respect, and understanding, and supports healing and recovery
  - **kia mōhio, kia mārama** – knowing where and how to access support
  - **mauri tau** – having easy access to support that recognizes and responds to their needs when they are affected by suicide

● Lived Experience Integrated into Leadership

The integration of lived experience of suicide into care systems is a critical step toward putting the patient at the center of those systems. "Lived experience" is provided by listening to and prioritizing the perspectives of those who receive services related to suicide prevention care, or who might receive such services in the future, or who might have received such services if systems were organized differently. Lived experience perspectives may come from people who have struggled with suicide concerns themselves, people who provide ongoing care for those with suicide risk, and people who have lost friends, family members, or colleagues to suicide. The core goal of **connecting** with people at risk of suicide can only be achieved if these perspectives are not only genuinely understood but also are put at the center of a system-level approach. This means designing systems around the needs of those at risk and ensuring that people with lived experience take an active role in developing, or "co-designing," systems of care.

In fostering a systems approach to suicide prevention, people with lived experience of suicide are given a significant role in decision-making bodies and are not just treated as an ancillary advisory group. A recent study of the co-production of services by service providers and users has emphasized that experience can only be drawn upon fully when service users are treated as fully respected members of the team, rather than people who should feel lucky to have their opinions heard. This means treating lived experience advocates and advisors in the same way that anyone else with specialized expert knowledge would be treated: Their hard work should be properly valued and they should be compensated financially for their time where appropriate, just like any other knowledge provider.[2]

● Restorative Just Culture

The ultimate negative outcome in suicide prevention care is the death of the person being cared for. The loss of a patient can be devastating for clinicians and can sometimes lead to long-term negative mental health outcomes. Compounding this natural reaction to the loss of human life are additional stressors that result from typical incident review approaches that follow in the wake of a patient death. These can add fears about legal and career consequences at what is already a difficult time for all those involved.

Traditional forms of incident review seek to allocate responsibility for adverse outcomes by identifying departures from standard clinical procedures or failures to assess risk correctly. Such processes are problematic for a number of reasons. Not only do they rely on incorrect assumptions about the ability of clinicians to accurately stratify risk (see Chapter 7), but the search for a linear account of "what went wrong" also fails to recognize the complexity of the environmental and historical circumstances that can contribute to a suicide attempt. Just as importantly, the goal of apportioning blame in post-incident reviews can lead to a culture of silence within an organization, and this presents a great obstacle to the aim of continuously improving care.

"People are not a problem to be solved or standardised:
they are the adaptive solution"
(Hollnagel et al., *From Safety-I to Safety-II: A White Paper.* 2015: 16–17)

When pursuing a systems approach to suicide prevention, it is important to recognize both that suicide can create "second victims" among the family and carers of the deceased, and that a culture of blame defeats learning. An alternative approach to post-incident review involves the creation of a "Restorative Just Culture"[3] in which the narrative shifts from asking "What is the root cause?" to "Whom has the suicide hurt?" and "What does each party need?" This approach acknowledges the loss and pain experienced by a range of stakeholders, including the deceased person themselves, as well as friends/family, the clinical care team, and even the broader community. This approach creates opportunities for healing and growth which often includes constructive critical feedback on systems without promoting a culture of pressure and mistrust. Learning thus becomes a way of restoratively processing suffering so as to diminish it in the future.

Restorative Just Culture

Incident review processes should align with principles of a Restorative Just Culture. These principles include:

- Identify and address harms, needs, and potential causes.
- Orient toward those in need (whether they are the consumer, their family or carer, or staff members, or the service and community – known as first, second, and third victims). Where possible, this includes engaging with all of these stakeholders.
- All parties are encouraged to recognize their role in the outcome and how they have been affected by it.
- All relevant stakeholders are included in rule development and processes for restoring trust.
- All discussions are based on shared/open dialog, active participation, and collaborative decision making.
- All discussions seek to identify and address the deeper, systemic issues that gave rise to the incident.
- The entire process is respectful to all parties.

(*Mental Health and Specialist Services, Post Incident Analysis: A Guide to Comprehensively Analyzing the Clinical Care Pathway*, November 2018)

D Best Practices, Policies, Pathways

Best practices for connecting, assessing, and responding to risk have been discussed in Chapters 5–7. Here we focus on the extension of best practices at a systems level.

● Pathways to Support Safety, Recovery, and Health

Utilizing defined service and intervention pathways offers an important tool for managing resource allocation issues. Criteria such as "current suicidal ideation nearly every day" or "suicidal ideation plus hospitalization in past year" can be a good starting point for placing people on a pathway involving more frequent assessment, more frequent contact, and more elaborate safety and contingency plans. Most health systems also allow people to be entered onto a pathway by clinician judgment/concern. This ensures that people who are expressing a certain kind of ideation and planning, or who have specific risk factors in their history, will rapidly receive the appropriate attention. However, it is important that entry into a pathway should not be based simply on a person's scores on a standardized scale, but rather on a well-considered formulation and identification of their risk status that takes account of their individual circumstances (see Chapter 6). Entry into a pathway should become a floor for defining base resource use but should not be treated as the primary driver of resource allocation, since risk stratification has not been proven to be valid and reliable. Resources in a pathway are best considered in terms of the factors that are driving a person's suicidality rather than the level of risk at which they are stratified.

● Codesign with Service Users and Families

An important development in suicide care systems has been an increasing focus on providing the most suitable healthcare context in the aftermath of a suicide attempt. This provides an example of the value to be found in working with service users and their families to design services that are built around their needs. Traditionally, those who have attempted suicide and those with pressing suicidal thoughts have been routed to the Emergency Department as a first point of healthcare contact. However, for someone suffering from the stressors that can precipitate a suicide attempt or thoughts of suicide, an emergency department can be a noisy, stressful environment that is both slow to respond and, in some countries, extremely expensive. In fact, recent research has suggested that those who receive Emergency Department care in these circumstances may be more likely to die by suicide later.[4,5]

In an attempt to resolve this mismatch between patient needs and treatment environment, policymakers and patient advocates have begun to explore the creation of dedicated spaces for those suffering from suicidal thoughts and behavior. These centers offer alternative destinations where people in crisis can be confident of receiving compassionate care in a comforting, less restrictive environment. One model for such centers is a Crisis Respite Center, which provides overnight support in a non-clinical environment by peers who have personal experience with suicidal ideation and attempts. Variations on this model may include professional counseling and nursing support, accommodation for support persons, and settings designed to reflect private homes. Initial research into the effectiveness of Respite Centers has been positive.[6] These centers are now being trialed in 14 US states and are being rolled out across Australia on a national level.[7]

● Continuous Quality Improvement

Adopting a health systems approach to care involves a commitment to ongoing improvement, not just a fixed-term program aiming at risk reduction over a year or two. The development of best practices and the structures to support them within given healthcare systems is a process of evolution, not an endpoint that can be reached definitively. Two important factors need to be balanced carefully in pursuing this evolution. On the one hand, practices and systems can only improve through close critical examination of what works and what does not. Learning takes place by constantly asking "What could be done better?" On the other hand, dealing with suicide concerns is already an emotionally difficult area of care due to the risk to life. When pursuing suicide reduction targets or working toward the goal of "perfect" or "zero defect" care, it is critical that the new frameworks are developed within a supportive working culture. Leaders need to establish a culture of zero tolerance for blaming and foster instead an understanding that suicide is traumatic for all those involved, including the care team.

For example, in many health systems engaged in suicide prevention quality improvement, even after the quality of the care provided by the organization improved, it was observed that gaps continued to exist in the crisis response system. It was customary to give people crisis line numbers, but a next step that could be taken was to integrate these services more fully within the healthcare system. For instance, by joining these services up with primary carers and emergency departments, it would become possible, with the permission of the caller, for a crisis line to directly access medical records and any previous safety planning information that had been drawn up in other care contexts.

Centers set up to respond to calls or texts also often have resources and infrastructure that can be used to further their goal of reducing suicide in other ways. These centers can provide contact after discharge from hospitals, as well as support for people in outpatient and community care during off hours. Crisis care is expanding in many regions to include planned and proactive structured follow-up, wellness checks, and general outreach. One of the most exciting advances in the field today is the growing number of partnerships between crisis intervention centers and health, behavioral health, and community service agencies. These institutional partnerships address continuity gaps that have been known about for years and are now finally being filled.

E **Engaged and Supported Workforce**

Programs for ongoing education in suicide prevention are critical to the implementation of health systems approaches to suicide prevention. Comprehensive suicide prevention training is not yet universal in mental health, nursing, or medical degree programs. While pre-professional education is improving, suicide prevention training will never be able to give a healthcare worker all they will ever need to know at a single point along their professional development trajectory. Evolutions in local and global standards of care, the complexity involved in working with people at risk of suicide, and the emotional challenges inherent in the task mean that there will always be a requirement for ongoing engagement, support, and encouragement. As such, most of the education that professionals will receive will be delivered while they are in the workforce. Health and human services organizations thus need to embrace this opportunity and their responsibility to ensure that this education serves the appropriate ends.

● **Shared Framework and Language**

One of the key goals for a health systems approach is to unite and inspire the workforce. A common framework within teams and across services lines and systems gives a clear message to those who are being looked after that the professionals they work with are part of a community that cares. Creating continuity at the systems level is not something that individual carers and clinicians can achieve alone. Culture is driven by common thought categories, language, and values, and these need to be spread at a high level. A coherent suicide-safer culture requires shared frameworks for connecting, assessing, responding, and extending the impact of care into the lives and support networks of the people being served.

Spreading and sustaining these frameworks and values relies on putting in place a system of education and support that explicitly conveys to trainees that the development of a health systems approach to care is a continuous process and that they will be supported in offering this care. The delivery system thus serves the twofold role of providing a medium for knowledge transfer while also creating and supporting a culture that is committed to preventing suicide. It needs to convey both content and process.

Application to Local Population/Culture

While the goal of a health systems approach to suicide prevention is to have a unified workforce with a common language and set of frameworks, it is also important to acknowledge that every local healthcare setting is a unique environment with unique individuals, culture, and patient and worker challenges. Training thus needs to communicate the shared knowledge that will join local cultures together into a unified system while also respecting differences and local requirements.

● Lived Experience Involvement in Workforce Education

The integration of lived experience perspectives into the design and development of healthcare systems is an essential feature of systems-based approaches (as discussed above). Training should also involve co-education with people who have received services in order to ensure that the patient perspective is fully integrated into the system of care.

● Sustainable Ongoing Learning

There is widespread consensus in the field that reduction in suicide rates will not occur with "one and done" training or by focusing only on credentialed mental health specialists. Suicide prevention education instead needs to expand both in terms of personnel targeted and also of the time horizon over which the training is delivered.

Members of the healthcare workforce who have the potential to prevent suicide are not limited to those employed in mental health settings or even those directly responsible for the provision of treatment and care. In order to provide coherent system-wide treatment, every individual working in health and community services needs training in suicide prevention. This includes medical providers and staff, case managers, non-clinical social workers, people who provide family case support, nurses, and group leaders. Depending on the context, the numbers involved can be daunting. Leaders thus need to find ways of onboarding people quickly into new cultural practices related to suicide prevention and safety.

Training must also be sustainable in the long term. In order to support a commitment to ongoing improvement, suicide prevention training needs to be delivered in a way that engages and motivates staff over time, and ensures that every new person in an organization can be brought quickly on board with suicide prevention culture and practices, while providing opportunities to interact with others. In particular, training that reaches out and puts individuals into contact with one another beyond their own immediate environments can draw attention to what they have in common and offer inspiring new perspectives. This in turn helps foster the system-wide view of prevention and care.

● Approaches to Workforce Education

An ideal workforce education model will thus be sustainable in economic terms, compatible with the highly demanding schedules of healthcare workers, and scalable to allow the provision of training to all members of large healthcare organizations. It should provide access to expert instruction, ongoing interaction with experts, and high-fidelity training content. It should also facilitate group interaction, the spread of learning within healthcare communities, and localized ownership of the training program.

Meeting all these goals at the same time is no easy task and common approaches to workforce education suffer from specific limitations.[8,9] Expert-led workshops and large group trainings are costly and difficult to schedule in healthcare and community service environments where time is at a premium. As such, they cannot be deployed in an ongoing and sustainable way at the healthcare system level. Train-the-trainer programs offer increased flexibility and provide a way to create local "champions" within a healthcare system; however, the fidelity of training content diminishes significantly when delivered by second-generation trainers[10] and such programs cannot offer everyone who takes part direct access to an expert. A national study of a train-the-trainer roll out of suicide prevention training, investigators found wide variability in adherence and competence among second-generation trainers.[11,12] Another study showed that this model is risky from a financial and impact perspective. Very few trainers prepared in this model go on to be productive trainers[13] – either because they move on to other roles or because they do not get enough practice to feel confident. Furthermore, such programs cannot offer everyone who takes part direct access to an expert.

Individual online learning ensures high fidelity to the material, and is affordable, flexible, and easily accessible. But working alone in front of a screen often leaves learners feeling as if they are just ticking boxes rather than being involved in systemic change. Intense time demands and the ability to multi-task makes it difficult to stay focused on modules. Further, dissemination research has shown that innovation spreads through interactions between colleagues and through networks of peers – such interaction is often missing from individually assigned modules.

Figure 10.2 Limitations of existing workforce education models

© 2018, SafeSide Prevention. Used with permission.

WORKFORCE EDUCATION MODELS

	ONLINE LEARNING	EXPERT WORKSHOPS	TRAIN-THE TRAINER	INPLACE® LEARNING
Expert instruction, high fidelity to content	✓	✓		✓
Ongoing interaction with expert				✓
Group interaction and experience		✓	✓	✓
Sustainable, repeatable for new staff education and refreshers	✓		Variable	✓
Local staff take ownership by leading groups			✓	✓

Blended learning approaches[14] are likely to be the best direction for scalable, sustainable workforce education, and engagement in suicide prevention. Blended learning takes advantage of the scalability of online learning but also judiciously adds time for group and instructor interaction. One such model in suicide prevention education is InPlace Learning, a workforce education approach developed by ARP. InPlace involves video-guided workshops[15] that teams work through together as a group – without need of an expert or second-generation trainer – followed by ongoing opportunities to engage with suicide prevention experts through Q&A videoconferences, online platforms, and brief microlearning refreshers.[16] Blended learning approaches are gaining traction in healthcare education and we expect more programs to adopt this multi-channel, multi-media approach.

KEY TAKEAWAYS

- The goal of a systems-based approach to suicide prevention is to work toward the aspirational goal of zero suicides in care.

- Explicitly adopting the terminology of "zero suicide" can be helpful, but is not required in order to pursue the aspirational goal. The decision concerning how to message about your health system's approach to suicide prevention must be made with sensitivity to the local context and culture.

- A health-system approach to suicide prevention involves implementing best practices and codesign of service pathways and policies, together with a commitment to continuous quality improvement. Lived experience perspectives and a non-blaming culture of continuous improvement are vital tools for achieving this end.

- A health systems approach to suicide prevention envisions the creation of shared language, frameworks, and practices across services within systems, and across systems within communities.

- Under a systems-based approach, education aims to unite and engage a diverse workforce serving diverse populations in diverse locations so that individuals can think, act, and communicate with a common set of principles and practices.

- Blended learning approaches are the future of workforce education, and key to scalable, sustainable workforce education.

10

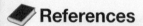

References

1   Hogan, M. F., & Grumet, J. G. (2016) Suicide prevention: An emerging priority for health care. *Health Affairs*, 35(6): 1084–90.

2   Soklaridis, S., de Bie, A., Cooper, R. B., et al. (2020) Co-producing psychiatric education with service user educators: A collective autobiographical case study of the meaning, ethics, and importance of payment. *Acad Psychiatry*, 44: 159–67. doi: 10.1007/s40596-019-01160-5.

3   Turner, K., Stapelberg, N. J., Sveticic, J., & Dekker, S. W. (2020) Inconvenient truths in suicide prevention: Why a Restorative Just Culture should be implemented alongside a Zero Suicide Framework. *Australian & New Zealand Journal of Psychiatry*, 54(6): 571–81.

4   Goldman-Mellor, S., Olfson, M., Lidon-Moyano, C., & Schoenbaum, M. (2019) Association of suicide and other mortality with emergency department presentation. *JAMA Netw Open*, 2(12): e1917571. doi: 10.1001/jamanetworkopen.2019.17571

5   Cerel, J., et al. (2006) Consumer and family experiences in the emergency department following a suicide attempt. *Journal of Psychiatric Practice*, 12(6): 341–47.

6   Shattell, M., Harris, B., Beavers, J., et al. (2014) A recovery-oriented alternative to hospital emergency departments for persons in emotional distress: "The living room". *Issues in Mental Health Nursing*, 35(1): 4–12. doi: 10.3109/01612840.2013.835012

7   www.health.nsw.gov.au/mentalhealth/resources/Pages/towards-zero.aspx

8   Pisani, A. R., et al. (2011) The Assessment and Management of Suicide Risk: State of Workshop Education. *Suicide Life Threat Behav*, 41(3): 255–76.

9   Pisani, A. R., Cross, W. F., Watts, A., & Conner, K. (2011) Evaluation of the Commitment to Living (CTL) Curriculum. *Crisis: The Journal of Crisis Intervention and Suicide Prevention*, 33(1): 30–38.

10 Cross, W. F., Chen, T., Schmeelk-Cone, K., et al. (2017) Trainer fidelity as a predictor of crisis counselors' behaviors with callers who express suicidal thoughts. *Psychiatr Serv*, 68(10): 1083–87.

11 Gould, M., Cross, W., Pisani, A. R., Munfakh, J. L., & Kleinman, M. (2013) Impact of applied suicide intervention skills training (ASIST) on national suicide training on the National Suicide Prevention Lifeline. *Suicide Life Threat Behav*, 43(6): 676–91. doi.org/10.1111/sltb.12049

12 Cross, W. F., Pisani, A. R., Schmeelk-Cone, K., et al. (2014) Measuring trainer fidelity in the transfer of suicide prevention training. *Crisis*, 35(3): 202–12. doi.org/10.1027/0227-5910/a000253

13 Cross, W., Cerulli, C., Richards, H., He, H. & Herrmann, J. (2010) Predicting dissemination of a disaster mental health "train-the-trainer" program. *Disaster Medicine and Public Health Preparedness*, 4(4): 339–43.

14 Rowe, M., Frantz, J., & Bozalek, V. (2012) The role of blended learning in the clinical education of healthcare students: A systematic review. *Medical Teacher*, 34(4): e216-e221.

15 Conner, K. R., Wood, J., Pisani, A. R., & Kemp, J. (2013) Evaluation of a suicide prevention training curriculum for substance abuse treatment providers based on Treatment Improvement Protocol Number 50. *J Subst Abuse Treat*, 44(1): 13–16. doi: 10.1016/j.jsat.2012.01.008. Epub 2012 Mar 13. PMID: 22417671; PMCID: PMC3640862.

16 Maggiulli, L., Donovan, S., Pisani, A. R., Aiello, J. & Russo, T. (2020) "Suicide prevention framework for youth services: Evaluation of a video-based learning program." Poster presentation at 32nd Annual Research and Policy Conference on Child, Adolescent, and Young Adult Behavioral Health.

SECTION 3
Special Topics: Medicolegal Considerations and Specific Populations

11 Medicolegal Risk Management

QUICK CHECK

A Introduction

Healthcare professionals manage medicolegal risk related to many different clinical issues and outcomes. Critical to risk management is an awareness of the duties we have as providers to our patients, and the steps that are considered standard practice for any particular clinical issue by similar health professionals. Included below are several considerations related to risk management and suicide-related outcomes:

- Legal systems and standards have considerable variability across countries, and this chapter addresses medicolegal issues related to suicide within the US context. Practitioners in the UK and other countries should familiarize themselves with any standards of clinical suicide-related practice. As in the USA, following standards of practice with attention to communication and documentation is the best way to protect both the patient's health and your own risk.

- Most healthcare professionals, even outside the field of mental or behavioral health, take care of patients at risk of suicide. Among patients who die by suicide, 60% had been seen by primary care, 40% in an emergency department, and 35% by a mental health professional in the several months prior to their death.[1] Health professionals in any discipline can be implicated in an adverse suicide-related outcome and the key is following best practice for one's given area of practice.

- In general, psychiatrists account for the lowest risk for malpractice suits of any medical specialists,[2] but suicide attempts and suicide deaths are among the more common reasons for malpractice suits for psychiatrists.

- Notably though, depending on the practice setting, suicide and suicidal behavior do not necessarily account for the majority of psychiatric malpractice claims: among claims one psychiatric malpractice insurance company received from 2006 to 2015 only 15% involved suicides or attempts. More than a third of the claims involved accusations of incorrect treatment, 20% were for medication-related issues, and 6% were for misdiagnosis.[3] Other reports do assert suicide accounts for the most common malpractice claim among psychiatric practices, specifically the failure to provide reasonable protection to a foreseeable outcome of patient suicide.[4]

- Avoiding suicide screening and risk assessment does **not** protect providers in the case of suicide or suicidal behavior. In many cases of suicide, the patient's risk was "latent" with no spontaneous expression of suicidal ideation or obvious sign of suicidal distress; other times clinicians may consciously or unconsciously avoid assessing suicide risk in their patients when clearer signals of risk are present, related to their own anxiety or other reasons such as lack of training or knowledge about standard practice related to suicide prevention. Therefore it is important to follow up on any clinical indications of suicide risk and follow best practices as outlined in this chapter and in greater detail in Section 2 of this book.

- In general, the plaintiff in a malpractice claim must show that the provider breached the duty of reasonable care or, in other words, was negligent. And, the plaintiff must show that he or she (or their loved one) was injured – either physically or mentally – by this negligence.

B **PRINCIPLES**

- By following recommended clinical care for patients during periods of suicide risk the provider can optimize patient outcomes and mitigate medicolegal risk.

- Standards of care for suicide prevention are touched on in this chapter and fully outlined in Chapters 6–9. These care standards should serve as clear guide posts for medicolegal risk management related to suicide.

- Learn the minimum recommended care steps for patients with suicide risk.

- Avoiding suicide screening and risk assessment does NOT protect providers in the event of suicide or suicidal behavior.

- Know who and when to screen for suicidal ideation.

- In behavioral health settings, suicide risk assessment should occur upon intake and should be updated and revised at key times throughout the care of patients. In primary care and other clinical settings, screening and assessment can occur either routinely or as indicated following your health system's policies and procedures.

- Stop using the out-of-date, ineffective "contracting for safety" and instead conduct Safety Planning Intervention.

- Document, document, document.

- If a patient does attempt or take their life, remember these are health outcomes that can occur even with appropriate care, like other health outcomes (e.g., myocardial infarction) that do still occur in some patients despite best care.

- In the event of patient suicide, follow the practical steps outlined in this chapter and also consider connecting with a community of clinicians who have experienced patient loss to suicide, to debrief and remain optimally healthy and active in clinical practice.

C **Brief Recommendations for Mitigating Risk for Patients and for Providers**

- **Know who and when to screen for suicidal ideation**: It is recommended practice (for example, in the current standards of The Joint Commission's National Patient Safety Goal NPSG 15.01.01) to **screen *all patients*** for suicidal

11

ideation in behavioral health settings. In other health settings (including in general medical/surgical hospitals, emergency departments and primary care settings in health systems), the requirement is to screen **as indicated**, such as when a patient presents with a primary mental health concern or condition or when there are other indicators of risk in the clinical history or current examination (e.g., recent job loss or other acute stressor and new symptoms of hopelessness, patient's affect atypical compared to baseline, or family reports concern about suicidal thoughts or preparations).

- **Know when to further assess suicide risk:** Another element of recommended practice is to more fully **assess suicide risk** when indicated, by an evidence-based process that goes beyond just focusing on the patient's current suicidal ideation.[5] The indications for conducting a suicide risk assessment include when suicidal ideation is present or when other clinical indicators point to possible increasing suicide risk (as discussed in Chapter 6).

- **It is ok that we cannot predict behavior or suicide, but we must follow standards of care** by identifying when suicide risk increases and providing key care steps. Science tells us there is no way for anyone – mental health professionals, primary care providers, or family/friends – to predict suicide in the near term (days to weeks). The key is to identify and address suicide risk to a feasible and reasonable extent, and document the steps taken to assess and mitigate suicide risk.

- **Managing medicolegal risk related to suicidal patients is similar to managing the risks related to other clinical scenarios**: The key is demonstration of **good faith effort** in identifying when patients' risk increases, and in providing the best care possible (including the steps in the National Action Alliance Recommended Practice document and The Joint Commission's 2019 Suicide Prevention National Patient Safety Goal, which include safety planning, lethal means counseling, referral, communication with family when possible, and following up with the patient even by telephone or other methods), and in documenting the process diligently.[6,7] These are currently considered the best care steps to employ in order to minimize the medicolegal risks associated with suicide.

- Applying the **ethical principles** of autonomy, non-maleficence, and beneficence to suicide preventive clinical care means using the most patient centered and least restrictive interventions.

Key Steps to Mitigate Risk for Both Patients and Providers

- Know who to screen (depends on clinical setting)
- Know when to screen for suicidal ideation (also depends on clinical setting)
- Know when to further assess with suicide risk assessment
- Use clinical judgment to screen and assess patients above and beyond what is "required" by policy or regulatory mandates
- Apply good faith effort to follow standards of care for patients who screen positive for either suicidal ideation screen or suicide risk assessment
- Stay patient centered in your approach and use the least restrictive measures as appropriate to the level of risk and the patient's specific foreseeable changes and options (outlined in Chapters 6–7).

Key Point: Prevention is Possible without Prediction.

There has been a conflating of prevention and prediction when it comes to suicide.

While predicting suicide in the near term is an area of intense interest in the suicide prevention scientific field, it is not currently possible to predict who will die by suicide or when. This does not mean prevention is not possible.

The same holds true for many other health-related causes of death, with a lack of precision for predicting mortality and timing. Just as cardiologists and primary care do not overly concern themselves with the lack of ability to predict which patients will die of heart disease or when, but remain focused on aggressively identifying and addressing risk factors in order to increase health outcomes (including mortality), the same can be done for preventing suicide. The key is monitoring risk and responding appropriately. Stick to recommended clinical assessment and care, and do so continuously over time while working with patients.

Just remember: Healthcare professionals are not expected to predict suicidal behavior or death, but are expected to practice and document reasonable steps according to accepted standards of practice. Practicing in an unduly defensive manner can paradoxically distract the clinician from staying the course with appropriate care. Fortunately, solid clinical care that is patient centered, supports the therapeutic alliance, and is consistent with current recommendations, **is** the best way to manage medicolegal risk.

11

D General Legal Considerations in Patient Care Related to Suicide

● Legal Standards

- Courts recognize that the prediction of future events and actions is not possible.
- However, physicians and other healthcare providers are held to standards of practice when clinical presentations indicating risk of suicide occur.

Required Elements for Plaintiffs in Malpractice Lawsuits

- A professional duty to the patient
- Breach of duty
- Injury caused by the breach
- Damages related to that injury

● The Issue of Foreseeability

- Am I expected to predict suicide? No but in the legal arena the issue is preventing a "reasonable foreseeability."
  - When is suicide a "foreseeable outcome"? Physicians can be held liable if the courts determine a patient's suicide was "foreseeable," and the physician's negligence in preventing the suicide was the actual and proximate cause of the patient's suicide.
  - See Chapter 6 for details about risk determination. If a patient has expressed a specific plan and an accessible and potentially lethal method with a stated time frame, along with other indicators of elevated suicide risk, this would likely be considered "reasonably foreseeable" unless other protective factors are present and documented.

● Typical Claims in a Wrongful Death Suit

The following are common claims in a wrongful death suit:

- Inadequate assessment: the provider failed to assess or document the risk of suicide.
- Failure to treat aggressively: the provider should have employed more intensive treatment or hospitalized the patient.
- Failure to refer for consultation: the provider should have referred the patient to a specialist.
- Failure to communicate between providers: two providers did not share enough information so that the primary provider did not realize the risk.

- Failure to reassess suicide risk: the provider failed to reassess the patient's risk and thus did not see that the risk had recurred or increased.
- Failure to follow patient safety protocols: in a hospital setting, the provider did not follow the policies and protocols related to suicide care, monitoring, or environmental inspection.

E **Standards of Care Related to Suicide Prevention**

Only in recent years has consensus truly been reached in the clinical arena of suicide prevention, establishing minimum standards of care in addressing patients at risk of suicide.[6]

Suicide Preventive Standards of Care
- The key to managing medicolegal risk for any clinical issue including suicide risk is to follow basic standards of care and document your assessment, clinical decision making, and care steps. (See Chapters 6–9.)
- Standards of care for suicide prevention have been evolving, reaching a new milestone of consensus in the field of suicide prevention. (See the Recommended Standards for People with Suicide Risk).[6]
- Notably, these recommended standards are quite consistent with the most recent Suicide Prevention National Patient Safety Goal standards by The Joint Commission, released 2019.[7]

11

One Approach: "Therapeutic Risk Management"
- Therapeutic risk management is one recommended approach to managing a patient who is suicidal.[8] Therapeutic risk management includes the following:
  o Conduct and document clinical risk
  o Augment clinical risk assessment with structured instruments to support clinical assessment. (See Appendix Resource List)
  o Determine the severity and timing of (stratify) the risk – e.g., whether the patient has intent and means; and whether the risk is imminent, near term, or long term
  o Conduct a Safety Plan Intervention with the patient and document
  o Develop a treatment plan for ongoing care and follow-up
  o Document every action taken and outcome achieved, including assessments, Safety Planning Intervention, lethal means counseling, follow-up disposition, and communication ongoing

● Evidence-based Care Examples

Know Who and When to Screen for Suicidal Ideation

- In the behavioral health setting, this includes **all** patients on a reasonably continuous basis throughout care.
- In primary care, mental health screening should be routine alongside all other regular general physical health screenings. Regulatory standards for primary care require screening for suicidal ideation as indicated including for patients with a psychiatric or substance use disorder.
- In emergency departments and other health settings, similar to primary care, regulatory standards require screening for suicidal ideation as indicated including for patients with a psychiatric or substance use disorder and when clinically indicated.

Continuous, Ongoing Suicide Risk Assessment

It is important to have a continuous filter for suicide risk assessment that continues beyond the initial assessment. On a periodic basis, if not with every relevant patient encounter, use your assessment of the patient's suicidal ideation, planning, access to lethal means, and intent to die versus live, alongside a continually updated assessment of the patient's risk and protective factors, and current psychosocial stressors/strengths and foreseeable changes to their circumstances. See Chapter 6 for the full guidance on risk assessment.

Safety Planning Intervention

- Developing a safety plan with the patient is considered one evidence-based way to provide standard of care for managing a suicidal patient. If the provider treats the patient ongoing, then continuing to work on the safety plan over time, and documenting each instance of updates, are highly recommended. Utilizing the Safety Planning Intervention along with other tools such as appropriate referral and ongoing communication has been found to reduce the likelihood of subsequent suicidal behavior in at-risk patients.[8]
- The rationale behind the Safety Planning Intervention is to work with the patient in developing individualized steps that he or she can take, both on their own, or in collaboration with loved ones and caregivers, to prevent acting on suicidal thoughts. There is research that shows reduction of subsequent suicide attempts by using safety planning in a high risk veteran population.[9]

- The following six steps of the Safety Planning Intervention should be written out by the patient or if using an application for safety planning on a mobile device, the patient should input their triggers and steps on the app:
  - o **Step 1. Warning signs**. Patients learn the indicators or red flags – the thoughts, feelings, and behaviors – that indicate the potential for suicidal action. Patients should describe in their own words these red flags – for example, "I am getting angry" and "I feel as if there's no use going on."
  - o **Step 2. Internal coping strategies**. Patients now list ways that they can cope with these feelings on their own. For example, "I think about my children."
  - o **Step 3. Distractions, activities, and positive environments**. Patients list ways for them to think about or do something else to take their minds off of the pressing distress without specifically asking for help. Examples could be, "I listen to this particular song or type of music" or "take a run through the park." They can make contact with a particular person as well without specifically asking for help at this step. The more specific and concrete these steps are, the better.
  - o **Step 4. People to ask for help**. Patients reach out to people who know about the patients' suicidal thoughts and are ready to help in any way they can, by listening and talking, spending time going somewhere or doing an activity together, or by expressing their support.
  - o **Step 5. Professionals and organizations to ask for help**. These include their therapist or psychiatrist and emergency resources such as crisis lines.
  - o **Step 6. Making the environment safe, clear of lethal means**. On their own or with the help of their loved ones, patients remove lethal means (firearms, medications, drugs, sharps, poisons) from their environment.
- Patient "suicide safety contracts" in which the patient agrees in writing not to act on suicidal thoughts, have been shown to be ineffective, and should not be used.[9]

Counseling on Access to Lethal Means

- Research has shown that access to means is a major risk factor for suicide and that reducing access to lethal means (even part of the time or temporarily for just the period of increased risk) reduces suicide risk.

- The most common methods used for suicide in the USA are firearms and hanging. In Asia the most common method is pesticides.
- Work with the patient and his or her family to limit the patient's access to firearms and potentially dangerous substances.
- There are training modules for learning how to provide Counseling on Access to Lethal Means ("CALM"). Ask your health system for training in suicide preventive care that includes safety planning and lethal means counseling education.
- Document all discussions with patient and family related to lethal means and about making the patient's environment as safe and clear of lethal means as possible.[10]

Collaborate with Other Professionals

- Do not hesitate to get consultation from other professionals, and to refer to or collaborate with mental health and substance abuse professionals, for follow-up care and therapy.
- There are specific types of treatment that are specifically suicide risk reducing, including DBT, CBT, CAMS or Attachment Based Family Therapy (ABFT). Consider referral to one of these forms of therapy, and document your efforts to make this type of referral. (See pp. 116–124 for more details about these recommended treatment modalities.)
- Document all consultations, referrals, and communication with other providers.

Hospitalization and Other Levels of Care

- New standards of care related to suicide prevention recommend using patient centered collaborative care, and the least restrictive methods possible. While many communities are not yet resourced with mobile crisis teams, crisis stabilization units, crisis homes, and peer support, these are all important options that can be appropriately utilized in lieu of the outdated model that only considers a binary decision: inpatient hospitalization versus outpatient care as usual. Even increasing the frequency of outpatient appointments and the use of between appointment communication through telephone, email, texting, and mail, are now considered suicide risk reducing measures.
- In instances of acute, high risk, involuntary hospitalization may be necessary.
  - o The standard practice criteria for involuntary hospitalization usually include the following:
    - The patient is a danger to self, or others related to their mental health condition OR

- The patient is gravely disabled, i.e., in danger of serious harm due to neglecting basic human needs (e.g., not taking food or hydration, or unable to provide basic clothing or shelter due to mental illness)

- Voluntary hospitalization is also an option for patients at moderate to high risk, especially when mitigating protective factors such as close follow-up, involvement of caring family members, or other forms of care are not available. Also when there are no clear solutions for the patient's foreseeable changes. (See Chapters 6–7 for details about treatment planning based on risk/protective factors and foreseeable changes.)

Communication with the Patient (and Family/Friends When Possible)

- Talk openly with the patient.
  - If risk factors for suicide are present (see Chapter 4), or if your clinical instincts detect a change in affect or behavior that may indicate depression or anxiety even in cases where mental health conditions have not been previously diagnosed (more than half of Americans with mental health conditions are not in treatment for them and may not have received a diagnosis), speak with them openly about possible signs and symptoms of mental health conditions.

  - Help the patient (and family when possible) to understand that mental health conditions are similar to most physical health conditions – they are multifactorial based on nature and nurture, genes, and environment. And that they can be managed over time just as physical health conditions can often be, with treatment, following up, and adjustments. Let your patient know that you will not give up on helping them feel better, that you are committed to their mental health getting back on track.

  - Ask if the patient is thinking about or planning suicide. Do not believe that bringing up suicide increases suicide risk. This is false – asking about their thoughts including of ending their life can provide relief especially if you are able to listen and provide non-judgmental support.[11] Find out how long their suicidal thoughts have been going on, if they can identify triggers, if they have made a plan or gathered means, and what their level of intent is for acting on the ideas.

  - Show the patient empathy and concern and let them know that, as their clinician, you want to understand and help them find ways to manage their mental health and their suicidal thoughts.

  - Ask for the patient's insights about what is working best along the way.

- It is important to empower the patient to take action and to stay on the side of living, rather than trying to be directive and commanding ("you must do this").
  - o Recognize that when people are feeling suicidal, ambivalence is a strong force at play – an internal battle between wanting to escape their pain and desperate seeming situation, and their healthier natural drive to live.
  - o Try to avoid the urge to find a quick solution to the patient's struggle. Practice active listening skills, ask open ended questions that give the patient the opportunity to become more insightful and activated to become well.
  - o Since you do not have any real power to compel the patient to do anything, giving commands is not the most effective strategy. Along these lines, there is no evidence for efficacy related to "No Suicide Contracts." Instead use safety planning.
  - o Also, be empathic and encourage the patient's motivation and self-efficacy ("I know you can do this. I'll stand by you. Together we will work on this until you feel better.").
  - o Document these communications with the patient, and any communications with family/friends.

 F | **Documentation**

● **Documentation Is Vital**

- It is critically important to review the recommended steps (Chapters 6–9), and document the steps you take to detect and assess risk, and to provide actions during the present visit as well as your follow-up care or contact.
- Also document your reason for believing the patient is not presently at acute risk, e.g., no plan/method/means gathered/intent, reasons for living, and which protective factors are strong.
- In sum, document each step of the decision-making process and every communication, oral or written, with the patient, family members and significant others, and other caregivers and medical professionals you've consulted with.
- Be as thorough and detailed in your documentation as possible.

Do's and Don'ts

- **Do** document:
    - Risk assessment: any screening or assessment instruments used, suicidal ideation, plans, intent, method, actions toward carrying out plan, discussion with patient about reasons for living/dying, prior risk and protective factors such as prior attempt, mental health conditions/deterioration, substance use, physical illness/pain, family history of suicide or mental health problems, prior trauma, exposure to others' suicidal behavior (celebrity, media or peer), access to lethal means (see Chapter 6).
    - Your risk assessment of level of present suicide risk, and a brief explanation of your reasoning.
    - Actions taken: develop a safety plan with the patient, counsel on lethal means present in the home, discuss with patient (and family) about follow-up with you and referral to a mental health professional, resources/referrals provided include 24/7 resources, such as the National Suicide Prevention Lifeline (1–800-273-TALK) and the Crisis Text Line text TALK to 741741.
    - Your rationale for the treatment plan including next steps.
    - Any consultation you've had with other experts/colleagues.
    - You should respond to family members who call with concerns about a patient with suicidal behaviors. Not responding because you do not have an authorization from the patient to release treatment information to the family member(s) is not a reason to communicate in ways that you are able.

- **Don't**:
    - Do not solely document "SI/no plan." Other factors are important to include, such as onset and characteristics of the suicidal thoughts, whether they have ever progressed to a plan, history of attempts, and other risk and protective factors.
    - Do not "contract for safety", i.e., ask the patient to promise not to attempt, not to act on suicidal thoughts. This practice, although common in the past, does not have evidence for reducing risk, is perceived negatively by patients, and does not afford medicolegal protection.
- Do not document **only** the first suicide risk assessment of a patient; risk assessment and documentation must be ongoing with monitoring and evaluation of suicide risk.
- Do not allow a patient with suicidal behaviors to be lost to follow-up care and communication by you or your clinic staff.

- For patients with recent suicidal behaviors or current high risk, do not neglect to document the clinical rationale for ordering a change in the level of patient supervision or care.
- Do not neglect to evaluate the safety of the environment for a patient with suicidal behaviors, e.g., accessibility of firearms and other weapons.
- For patients determined to be at high risk presently, do not forget to ensure that during transport within the hospital or during transitions to other units or facilities, the same level of monitoring is continued.

G | **After a Patient Suicide**

It can be challenging on multiple levels to experience the death of a patient by suicide.[12] Make sure to acknowledge your reactions, debrief with trusted colleagues, and consider the following recommended steps.[13] Consider the recommended steps in the following box which include communicating with trusted peers, mentors, risk management, and your insurance company, as well as offering to meet with the patient's family.

Steps to Take Following Patient Suicide

- Contact your insurance company and your health system's risk management team immediately.
- Reach out to the decedent's family/survivors.
- While anxiety provoking and clinical boundaries still need to be maintained after death, it is recommended to meet with the family to support them in their grief and to answer questions when possible. It is not only ok, but it is recommended in many instances to offer a meeting with surviving family members. Helping them process their grief and sharing limited information can be a positive step for all, and can mitigate against risk. Discuss the details of the situation with a trusted colleague, suicide expert, and risk management.
- Refer family members for grief counseling if appropriate.
- It is reasonable to relieve surviving family of any financial obligations, where applicable.
- Do not alter the medical record.
- If a patient suicide occurs in a training setting, then engage training program leadership in a compassionate, appropriate debriefing process for all trainees, faculty, and other health disciplines such as nurses who were involved.[14]

KEY TAKEAWAYS

a. By following the current recommended clinical care standards, the health professional optimizes patient outcomes and mitigates medicolegal risk.

b. Clinicians' most important guide for managing medicolegal risk is learning and following current recommended care and documenting well.

c. Avoiding suicide screening and risk assessment does **not** protect providers in the event of suicide or suicidal behavior, even when providing care via telehealth or telemedicine services.

d. "Contracting for safety" is no longer considered useful either for improving patient care nor for risk mitigation. The Safety Planning Intervention in concert with lethal means counseling, appropriate referral, ongoing follow-up and communication does show evidence for reducing risk and is a recommended practice across many health settings.

e. If a patient does attempt or take their life, remember suicide is a health outcome that can occur even with appropriate care, like other complex health outcomes (e.g., myocardial infarction). These untoward outcomes occur in some patients despite best care.

f. In the event of a patient loss to suicide, steady yourself and follow the practical steps outlined in this chapter and in Chapter 17. Consider connecting with a community of clinicians who have experienced patient loss to suicide, to debrief and remain optimally healthy and active in clinical practice.

11

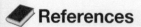

References

1   Luoma, J. B., Martin, C. E., & Peason, J. L. (2002) Contact with mental health and primary care providers before suicide: A review of the evidence. *Am J Psychiatry*, 159(6): 909–16.

2   Jena, A. B., Seabury, S., Lakdawalla, D., & Chandra, A. (2011) Malpractice risk according to physician specialty. *N Engl J Med*, 365: 629–36.

3   Professional Risk Management Services. (2016) New Cause of Loss Data from the Psychiatrists' Program. Retrieved from www.prms.com/prms-blog/articles/2016/february/new-cause-of-loss-data-from-the-psychiatrists-program/

4   Sher, L. (2014) Suicide medical malpractice: an educational overview. *International Journal of Adolescent Medicine and Health*, 27(2): 203–6. Retrieved 19 Nov. 2019, from doi: 10.1515/ijamh-2015-5012

5   Patient Safety & Quality Healthcare. (2019) TJC Clarifies Suicide Risk NPSG Requirements. Retrieved from www.psqh.com/news/tjc-clarifies-suicide-risk-npsg-requirements/

6   National Action Alliance for Suicide Prevention: Transforming Health Systems Initiative Work Group. (2018) Recommended Standard Care for People with Suicide Risk: Making Health Care Suicide Safe. Retrieved from theactionalliance.org/sites/default/files/action_alliance_recommended_standard_care_final.pdf

7   The Joint Commission. (2019) Suicide Prevention Portal. Retrieved from www.jointcommission.org/topics/suicide_prevention_portal.aspx

8   Matarazzo, B. B., Homaifar, B. Y., & Wortzel, H. S. (2014) Therapeutic risk management of the suicidal patient: Safety planning. *J Psychiatr Pract*, 20(3): 220–24. doi: 10.1097/01.pra.0000450321.06612.7a

9   Stanley, B., Brown, G. K., Brenner, L. A., et al. (2018) Comparison of the safety planning intervention with follow-up vs usual care of suicidal patients treated in the emergency department. *JAMA Psychiatry*, 75(9): 894–900. doi: 10.1001/jamapsychiatry.2018.1776

10 Suicide Prevention Resource Center. (2018) CALM: Counseling on Access to Lethal Means. Retrieved from www.sprc.org/resources-programs/calm-counseling-access-lethal-means

11 Gould, M. S., Marrocco, F. A., Kleinman, M., et al. (2005) Evaluating iatrogenic risk of youth suicide screening programs: A randomized controlled trial. *JAMA*, 293(13): 1635–43. doi: 10.1001/jama.293.13.1635

12 Gutin, N. (2019) Losing a patient to suicide: Navigating the aftermath. *Current Psychiatry*, 18(11): 17–24.

13 Gitlin, M. (1999) A psychiatrist's reaction to a patient's suicide. *Am J Psychiatry*, 156(10): 1630–34.

14 Coverdale, J. H., Roberts, L. W., & Louie, A. K. (2007) Encountering patient suicide: emotional responses, ethics, and implications for training programs. *Acad Psychiatry*, 31(5): 329–32.

12

The Role of Culture and Societal Factors

QUICK CHECK

A PRINCIPLES

- Suicide rates vary widely across various cultures and geographically distinct groups.

- A complex health outcome influenced by many factors, suicide most often occurs when internal (biological, psychological, cognitive, genetic) and external (psychosocial stressors, family dynamics, and sociocultural factors) risk factors converge.

- Gaps in research related to culture and suicide risk notwithstanding, cultural factors are generally thought to influence the suicide risk of a population.

- Experiences of racism and marginalization impact mental health outcomes negatively. Research on the suicide risk factors of indigenous, marginalized, and minority populations are much needed areas for further investigation.

- Beliefs held by an individual or an entire group impact behavioral norms and attitudes toward mental health, disclosure of distress, and help seeking.

- When suicide is viewed as a normalized behavior either in general or in response to a stressor such as bullying, suicide risk can increase for that population.

- When struggles are viewed as a normal part of the human condition, and help seeking, leaning on social support, and mental health treatment are viewed as acceptable or even signs of strength, suicide rates have been shown to decrease.

- Availability and attitudes toward particular lethal means also impact suicide rates.

- National and regional suicide prevention programs have proven effective in addressing culture, stigma, help seeking, and suicide rates.

 Introduction

Cultural factors including conscious and unconscious beliefs and attitudes have an influence on suicide risk for individuals, families, and populations. A body of research demonstrates that suicide risk draws on multiple risk and protective factors at the individual and environmental levels. By understanding how particular beliefs and stigma may impact suicide risk, healthcare professionals can communicate more effectively with patients from different cultural backgrounds for the purpose of both risk assessment and patient care. For example, eliciting the patient's perspectives about particular life challenges, about mental healthcare, and even about suicide itself, can be useful in engaging the patient in both self-care and treatment planning.

Examples: Eliciting beliefs can improve communication

Eliciting patients' thoughts and beliefs about their struggles, about mental healthcare, and even about suicide itself, can be useful in engaging the patient in both self-care strategies and treatment planning.

For example:

1. If the patient identifies a belief about failures equating to worthlessness or deserving to die, this could be a clinical target for psychotherapy and treatment.

2. If their parents or community espoused the belief that "only crazy people see psychiatrists," this could be an opportunity for psychoeducation and reframing. An example of successful reframing could include, "Many successful people use therapy/treatment to sharpen their mental clarity and to optimize their health."

3. If a male patient expresses a view that "men don't get therapy," that provides an opportunity for targeted education and intervention to help the patient understand that many men do engage in mental health treatment to the benefit of their mental **and** physical health and their ability to fulfill roles at home and/or work.

4. If patients learned a dichotomous or rigid way of judging their actions or circumstances, as part of family, religious, or cultural norms, flexibility and a growth mindset could be part of the treatment goals. For example, "Not everything falls into the right versus wrong or success versus failure categories. Life is full of unexpected hardships or mistakes, and I can learn and grow from them and through them."

5. If the patient has lost a family member to suicide and they had thought that it meant they are destined to take their own life, this would be a very important target for psychoeducation and possible further inquiry about this belief. For example, while genetics and family history do contribute risk and protective factors for suicide, genes do not determine destiny and most risk can be mitigated through a variety of strategies like identifying their own triggers, using a safety plan, getting treatment for mental health conditions, and learning how to talk with a partner about life struggles. Just as they would take extra care if they knew they had family members who died young of heart disease, the same is true for suicide, enhancing and their ability to protect themselves and change potential negative clinical outcomes.

12

C   The Role of Cultural and Societal Factors

Suicide cuts across all racial/ethnic, geographical, occupational, gender, and age groups, however there are particular groups with higher rates of suicide. In the USA the demographic groups with the highest rates include middle-aged and older White males, and young American Indian males. Other groups such as Black children and adolescents, Latinx female adolescents and Asian American youth have higher rates of attempts, and this also warrants attention. Geographical differences, for example with the Rocky Mountain states and Alaska having the highest rates of suicide in the USA, may stem more from cultural values related to stoicism and self-sufficiency, access to mental healthcare, and the availability of lethal means such as firearms and opioids. The CDC's most recent analysis of occupational groups finds agricultural, farming, construction, first responder, law enforcement, healthcare, and entertainment industries with higher rates of suicide.

Elements of Culture/Environment that Can Impact Population Suicide Risk

- Beliefs and attitudes about distress, need for support, and self-sufficiency
- Attitudes toward mental health conditions, experiences, symptoms, distress
- Attitudes toward mental healthcare
- Accessibility and affordability of mental healthcare
- Knowledge about mental health treatment options, risks, and benefits
- Stigma surrounding mental health distress and need for help
- Rates of engaging in mental healthcare
- Social structures that promote interpersonal connectedness
- Family, faith, or cultural values that incorporate human need for attachment, relational bonds, forgiveness, and support
- Accessibility of lethal means
- Media practices related to reporting on suicide
- Discriminatory policies and practices related to mental health conditions and addiction
- Attitudes toward suicide
- Population density (higher density areas generally have lower suicide rates than lower density areas)
- Current and historical trauma

Suicide Rates Vary Significantly between Populations

Differences in suicide rates between groups, nations, and cultures are large. Beliefs related to mental health, stigma surrounding life struggles, attitudes toward help seeking, access to lethal means, and strategic suicide prevention efforts all play a role in a population's risk for or protection from suicide. Surveillance of suicide is also highly variable between countries so that reported rates may be gross underestimates of true rates. (See Figure 1.7 for details of variability in suicide data across countries).

As of 2021, 40 countries have national suicide prevention strategies, and several of these have seen reductions in their nation's suicide rate.[1] The USA is one of few nations which has seen a consistently rising suicide rate over the past two decades, increasing a staggering 35% overall from 1999 to 2018 with the first decrease by 2.1% from 2018 to 2019. Many European countries such as those in the UK have seen fairly consistent rates over recent years, and other countries such as Australia, Finland, Denmark, Norway, South Korea, and Japan, which have more progressively implemented national suicide prevention plans, have seen reductions in suicide rates.

For a view of the suicide rate trends over time, please see https://ourworldindata .org/suicide for interactive graphs sourced from WHO data, that show changes in countries' suicide rates over recent decades.

The culture and beliefs of a population influence not only risk but protective factors as well. For example, communities and cultures where interpersonal connectedness is strong via family, peer, and community relationships, tend to have lower risk of suicide, especially when the prevailing culture promotes openness about mental health experiences and help seeking.

How Does Culture Impact Suicide?

● Stigma and Seeking Help

Numerous studies demonstrate a relationship between population suicide rates and beliefs about mental health and help seeking. A Dutch study of stigma and help seeking compared the Flemish region of Belgium, in which the suicide rate is among the highest in the world, to the Netherlands, in which the suicide rate is much lower. The study showed that in the Netherlands, people had more positive attitudes toward help seeking and experienced less self-stigma and shame about mental health problems. Conversely, a sense of shame and negative attitudes toward help seeking existed in the Flemish community. Flemish women were more reticent to seek professional or informal help, and Flemish men received less help for psychological problems than Dutch men.[3] There is a strong correlation between stigma surrounding help seeking and rates of suicide.

Figure 12.1 Suicide rates by state in the USA

Within countries, suicide rates also vary significantly. For example, in the USA, the suicide rates in Rocky Mountain states such as Montana and Wyoming and other states like Alaska are in the range of 25–29 per 100,000 per year, whereas in states such as New York and Maryland, rates are 6–9 per 100,000 per year. Similar differences in smaller regions county to county within a given state exist, likely reflecting differences in beliefs and culture that impact stigma and help seeking, population density and interpersonal connectivity, accessibility of healthcare including mental healthcare, and access to lethal means such as firearms availability.[2]

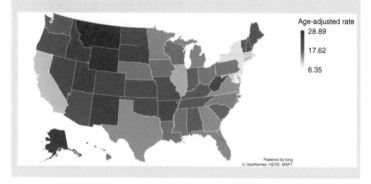

Age-adjusted rate
28.89
17.62
6.35

Powered by bing
© GeoNames, HERE, MSFT

Social norms surrounding aspects of identity such as gender and occupation also suggest a strong influence on stigma related to mental health and help seeking. For example, particular groups such as American men, minority and marginalized communities, farmers, law enforcement, physicians and other health professionals, among other demographic and occupational groups, tend to be less likely to seek care from mental health professionals. Many prefer to turn to peers, friends, faith leaders, and primary care providers. Therefore efforts to educate the lay public, including so called "gatekeeper training", i.e., suicide prevention training of faith leaders, parents, teachers, and law enforcement, have an important role in equipping community members to have caring, supportive conversations, and how to lead at-risk individuals to professional help. Primary care providers also play a pivotal role since many people are willing to raise mental health concerns with their primary care provider. And far more individuals who attempt or die by suicide have seen a primary care provider than a mental health provider, in the weeks preceding their attempt or death.

● **When Suicide Is Viewed as Acceptable**

In rare instances, when suicide is viewed as a culturally acceptable method of coping or self-expression, this may lower the barrier to moving from thought to action for a suicidal individual, and creates a significant cultural risk factor, especially for particular individuals who have other suicide risk factors.

Historical Japanese Example of Beliefs about Suicide

One example of a belief that viewed suicide in a way that made it acceptable is the traditional Japanese practice of harakiri or seppuku from twelfth century samurai culture. This gruesome form of self-disembowelment was seen as an expression of atonement for defeat, protest of a superior's decision, or extreme respect. The lore is that when a Japanese emperor died in 1912, his leading general performed harakiri as an act of respect for the leader. This was one prominent example among many of this practice of extreme self-sacrifice to express honor and respect to a supreme authority figure. While the practice of harakiri is rare in modern day Japan, cultural threads of this notion are still present and can exert influence, especially if an individual is becoming at risk for suicide for other individual reasons (multifactorial deterioration in mental health, genetic loading for mood or psychotic disorder or for suicide, prior history of early adverse events, etc.).

Key Point

In any culture, when media portrays suicide in sensational ways including showing suicide as an effective pathway for being memorialized as a hero or as a pathway for revenge, this can increase risk. These portrayals may have a similar effect to cultures that view suicide as a method for obtaining honor, power, or revenge.

12

● **Suicide Methods in Culture**

Culture and societal norms can play an important role in the suicide risk and rates of a population by the way specific methods for suicide are viewed and addressed. In some cultures, there are very particular traditional methods of suicide that send a specific message – the Japanese tradition of harakiri, as discussed above, is undoubtedly the most famous, and these historically contextualized views of suicide can exert an influence even into modern times.

Science is very clear that suicide rates of a population are impacted by the general availability and accessibility of lethal means. Case examples include the firearm-oriented culture of many regions in the USA alongside research that demonstrates that households with firearms have higher rates of firearm suicide. The precipitous rise in the availability of opioids, especially highly lethal versions such as fentanyl in many parts of the USA, has likely impacted population suicide rates in those areas. Both firearms and opioids are highly available lethal means which have likely played a role in the rise in US suicide rates during the two decades of the twenty-first century.

Similarly, pesticides have been a leading method of suicide in many Asian countries related to their availability and accessibility in many households. When public health efforts were taken to educate pesticide vendors and community members about the importance of safe storage, and when legislative efforts changed the availability of particularly lethal pesticides, the suicide rates decreased in those regions of the world.[4]

One historical example of the link between availability of means and suicide rates occurred in the second half of twentieth century England with the detoxification of domestic gas, occurring as a natural result of new forms of energy being utilized in place of coal. Not only did the rate of suicide by gas inhalation decrease significantly, but the overall rate of suicide in England decreased by 40%. This is one of several naturalistic studies demonstrating the critical role of lethal means reduction in suicide prevention, also highlighting the consistent finding that the majority of suicidal people **do not** necessarily switch to a different method if the original method is not accessible.[5]

● Racism and Mental Health

Experiences of racial discrimination are common among many minorities and indigenous populations. Research on the effects of racial trauma show a clear relationship between experiences with discrimination, violence, assault, or harassment and outcomes such as depression, PTSD, anxiety, addiction, and other serious mental health conditions. Combined with other risk factors, trauma can also increase risk of suicide. Shame is a common experience of many victims, even when they have done nothing wrong. Additionally, minority communities experience many ongoing injustices such as microaggressions, disparities in educational opportunities, inadequate access to effective, culturally competent healthcare, and economic disparities, all on top of generations of trauma. All of these systemic injustices contribute to negative mental health outcomes. As with many experiences of injustice or trauma, an individual's health impact and response rely on not just the current experience, severity, and circumstance, but occurs on a complex backdrop of the individual's prior experiences, prior trauma, and mental health history.

Focus on Black American Youth Suicide

As an example of the need to focus more effort on cultural factors unique to particular minority populations, without much attention until now, the suicide rate among Black youth in the USA has been increasing faster than any other racial/ethnic group in the USA. Although Black youth have historically not been considered at high risk for suicide or suicidal behaviors, current trends demonstrate the contrary.[6] Albeit rising from a low base rate, Black youth under 13 years old have had concerning trends with increases in suicidal behavior and death, now being twice as likely to die by suicide as their White counterparts. Self-reported suicide attempts have increased by 73% for Black male and female adolescents over two decades. This is while self-reported suicidal thoughts and plans have decreased, pointing to a need to examine why they may be going straight to attempts, or not able to express ideation or plans. Meanwhile, Black adolescents are significantly less likely to receive care for depression – a major risk factor for suicide – with experts identifying pervasive structural inequities, social determinants of health, stigma, and mistrust of healthcare providers creating daunting barriers to treatment.

In a US Congressional Black Caucus Emergency Task Force on Black Youth Suicide a group of experts convened in 2019 to explore what is and is not known about the societal, cultural, health, educational, and economic factors and disparities that may be contributing to the increases in youth Black suicide. Their report, "Ring the Alarm: The Crisis of Black Youth Suicide in America", documents a dearth of research to understand these trends, even pointing to a lack of understanding about risk factors and warning signs of suicide in Black American youth.[7]

The recommendations of the Task Force broadly include:

1. Increased research into topics relating to Black youth mental health and suicide through federal funding including for Black researchers who are focused on these topics.
2. Demonstrate and promote evidence-based interventions and best practices for clinicians, school personnel, teachers, parents, and others who interact with Black youth.

Specific ideas for addressing cultural barriers with the goal of advancing suicide prevention for Black youth include:

1. Establish training academies for school-based personnel and mental health providers on how to recognize signs of depression, suicidal behaviors, and other mental health problems.

2. Fund the development of a model curriculum for administrators, teachers, other school personnel, parents, and community-based organizations and around mental health and suicide. Such a curriculum must include training in anti-bias, anti-oppressive, and gender equity practices.

3. Develop culturally effective guidelines for national suicide and mental health hotlines and organizations relating to Black youth.

4. Identify and promote best and promising practices for increasing the pipeline of social workers and other mental health providers to address the dearth of school-based personnel who can address the mental health needs of Black students, with the goal of placing a proportionate number of social workers and other mental health providers in each school relative to the student body population.

5. Develop a screening tool for use by providers across healthcare professionals and institutions relating to suicidal thoughts, ideation, and self-harm, as well as a protocol on how to treat and connect Black youth to care.

KEY TAKEAWAYS

a. Suicide rates vary widely across various cultures and geographically distinct groups.

b. Many factors, including cultural attitudes, beliefs, and experiences impact the suicide risk of a population.

c. Beliefs held by an individual or an entire group impact behavioral norms and attitudes toward mental health, disclosure of distress, and help seeking.

d. More research is needed to better understand the specific risk and protective factors for many demographic groups, particular minority populations where research is especially lacking.

e. When struggles are viewed as a normal part of the human condition, and help seeking, interpersonal connectedness, and mental health treatment are viewed as signs of strength, suicide rates can decrease.

f. Availability and attitudes toward a particular lethal means impact suicide rates of a population. Making lethal means for suicide less accessible both for whole populations as well as for an individual during a period of risk is a critical part of preventing suicide.

g. National and regional suicide prevention programs have proven effective in addressing culture, stigma, help seeking, and suicide rates.

References

1   **National Suicide Prevention Strategies: Progress, Examples and Indicators. (2018)** Geneva: World Health Organization. License: CC BY-NC-SA 3.0 IGO. Retrieved from www.who.int/health-topics/suicide#tab=tab_1

2   **Centers for Disease Control and Prevention. (2018)** Mortality in the United States, 2017. Retrieved from www.cdc.gov/nchs/products/databriefs/db328.htm.

3   **Reynders, A., Kerkhof, J. F. M., Molenberghs, G., & Van Audenhove, C. (2015)** Help-seeking, stigma and attitudes of people with and without a suicidal past. A comparison between a low and a high suicide rate country. *J Affect Disord*, 178(1): 5–11.

4   **Gunnell, D., Knipe, D., Chang, S., et al. (2017)** Prevention of suicide with regulations aimed at restricting access to highly hazardous pesticides: A systematic review of the international evidence. *Lancet Glob Health*, 5(10): e1026-e1037.

5   **Kreitman, N. (1976)** The coal gas story: United Kingdom suicide rates 1960–71. *Brit J Prev Soc Med*, 30: 86–93.

6   **Bridge, J. A., Horowitz, L. M., & Fontanella, C. A., et al. (2018)** Age-related racial disparity in suicide rates among US youths from 2001 through 2015. *JAMA Pediatrics*, 172(7): 697.

7   **Emergency Task Force on Black Youth Suicide and Mental Health. (2019)** Ring the Alarm: The Crisis of Black Youth Suicide in America. Retrieved from watsoncoleman.house.gov/uploadedfiles/full_taskforce_report.pdf

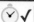

13

Youth and Adolescents

 QUICK CHECK

A Introduction: Youth Suicide, a Global Public Health Crisis

Suicide among youth is a major public health concern globally. According to the WHO, suicide is the second leading cause of death in the world for 10–29-year-olds. It is important to recognize that young people are more likely to die by suicide than by any other single medical illness, underscoring the need for increased emphasis on medical education regarding suicide and the potential lifesaving impact of identification and effective care for youths with elevated suicide risk. Because suicidal ideation and behavior tend to have their first onsets during adolescence, this developmental period may offer an important window of opportunity to prevent the development of suicidal thoughts and behaviors, which lead to elevated risk of premature death, mental health and functioning problems, and psychological pain and distress.

Among the 40 countries with national suicide prevention plans, many address youth suicide utilizing a public health approach that includes universal education about mental health, suicide risk factors, and warning signs, and how to change culture and stigma particularly surrounding help seeking. Additionally, targeted efforts are underway to augment peer support training, engage high risk populations, and better prepare health professionals and systems to appropriately identify and care for youth at risk for suicide.

 PRINCIPLES

- Youth suicide is a global public health crisis warranting major investments and actions commensurate with its morbidity and mortality toll.

- Youth suicide takes more lives in the USA than all other medical causes of death together.

- Suicide risk factors in youth include family, school, and peer interactions in addition to the universal risk factors for all ages such as unaddressed mental health conditions, lethal means availability, and genetics.

- The clinical identification and management of emerging mental health conditions in youth is a critical aspect of youth suicide prevention.

- Health professionals can play an important role in dispelling myths surrounding medications as well as utilizing or advocating for all effective treatment modalities.

- Social media plays a significant role in the mental health and suicide risk for some youth. Incorporating social media utilization and its particular impact on an individual into clinical assessment and treatment planning is recommended.

- Youth are more susceptible to suicide contagion than adults, therefore mitigating suicide exposure among youth is a key prevention strategy.

- Suicide screening and assessment for youth are recommended with recently validated tools.

- It is imperative for pediatricians, parents, school personnel, and peers to all play a role to prevent youth suicide.

 Scope of the Problem and Trends

Suicide is rare in children under 13 years old, however during the adolescent years rates increase and the gender differential gap begins and widens into adulthood.

While rates are lower in youth than in middle and older age groups in most high-income countries (in the USA, American Indians are one exception), any loss of life early to a preventable cause like suicide is tragic and warrants effort and attention.

217

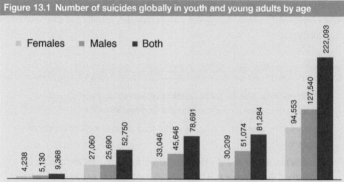

Figure 13.1 Number of suicides globally in youth and young adults by age

Legend: Females | Males | Both

	Females	Males	Both
10–14 yrs	4,238	5,130	9,368
15–19 yrs	27,060	25,690	52,750
20–24 yrs	33,046	45,646	78,691
25–29 yrs	30,209	51,074	81,284
10–29 yrs	94,553	127,540	222,093

● Spotlight on Youth Suicide in the USA

As is the case globally, suicide is the second leading cause of death for youth aged 15–24 in the USA. Only unintentional injuries, including car accidents and drug overdoses, take more young American lives every year.

- Approximately one in six teenagers in the USA seriously considers suicide over a 12-month period.[3]

- In the USA an estimated 100–200 youth attempt suicide for every youth death by suicide. The suffering and trauma that suicidal behavior encompasses, for the young person, their parents, siblings, peers, and for schools and others is enormous. In the USA the K-12 educational system has become increasingly involved in suicide prevention of youth via school suicide prevention policies, mandatory suicide prevention training of teachers and staff, and procedures for handling suicidal students and re-entry to school after inpatient or intensive mental health treatment for suicide attempts.

- Girls are more likely to attempt suicide than boys, but as with the adult population, boys are more likely to die by suicide than girls. A 2019 study of the 40-year youth suicide trends in the USA found that youth suicide rates increased from 1975 to 1992, decreased from 1992–2007, and have been

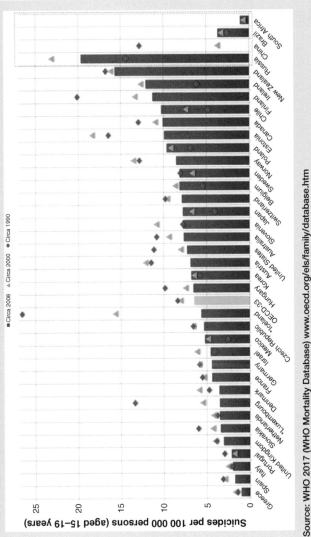

Figure 13.2 Teenage suicide (15–19 years) by country per WHO Mortality Database

Trends are shown for each country, e.g., blue and green markers above the red bar indicate a decrease in teen suicide rates over nearly two decades.[1]

Source: WHO 2017 (WHO Mortality Database) www.oecd.org/els/family/database.htm

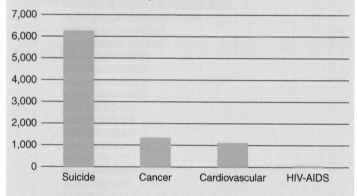

Figure 13.3 Suicide is a leading cause of adolescent and young adult death in the USA

For youth aged 15–24 in the USA, suicide takes more lives than the other leading health-related causes of death in youth combined.[2]

Source: National Vital Statistics Report, Deaths: Final Data for 2017, www.cdc
.gobe/nchs/data_access/Vitalstatsonline.htm

increasing from 2007 to 2016.[4] In fact a CDC report on US youth suicide trends published in 2020 found the suicide rate among adolescents and young adults aged 10–24 in the USA increased an astounding 57.4% from 6.8 per 100,000 in 2007 to 10.7 in 2018.[5] Additionally the gender gap is narrowing especially for youth aged 10–14 years old. Among youth suicide decedents, the more lethal method of suffocation/hanging has been rising particularly for girls over this past decade.

• Girls between the ages of 15 and 19 years old attempt suicide at twice the rate of boys, yet boys' suicide rate which was three times the rate of girls, has more recently been found to be two times higher, indicating a narrowing of the gender gap in American youth suicide rates, with both genders' rates on the rise.[4]

D Suicide Risk Factors Specific to Youth

Many suicide risk factors – notably depression and other mental health deterioration including substance abuse – are as true for adolescents as they are for adults. There are however more young suicide decedents for whom the deterioration in mental health may have been undetected due to their early life stage and less time and history to have noted the signs of a mental health condition. Changes in mental health tend to be more challenging to recognize during the adolescent years related to actual variability in clinical presentations during youth as well as difficulty many parents have differentiating between "normal teen angst" and clinically significant symptoms.

Behaviors in the Home Matter

Research from the Family Acceptance Project led by Dr. Caitlin Ryan found specific behaviors in the home contribute to serious health outcomes for LGBTQ youth. Supportive versus rejecting behaviors in the home were associated with significantly different health-, mental health-, and suicide-related outcomes. Rejecting behaviors such as parents or other family members telling the child they are ashamed of them, blaming the child when peers mistreat them because of their LGBTQ identity or gender expression, not using the name or pronoun that matches the child's gender identity, or causing them to leave home because they are LGBTQ were associated with serious health outcomes including depression, suicidal thoughts and attempts, substance use, and HIV/AIDS. The more of these behaviors that parents and family members do, the greater the risk to the LGBTQ child's health, whereas supporting behaviors such as telling the child you love them and expressing affection when the child talks about being LGBTQ, supporting their gender expression, requiring other family members to treat the child with respect, and speaking with faith leaders and others to help them become supportive of LGBTQ people, are all associated with reductions in the child's likelihood of experiencing suicidal thoughts, attempts, and substance use problems. Please visit https://familyproject.sfsu.edu/ to learn more and request posters for your clinic that provide this critically important information for parents.[9]

There are also particular risk factors that are more critical in youth suicide risk than for adults: these include child–parent conflict and negative family dynamics, parental substance use or mental illness, peer conflict, LGBTQ rejection by parents and others, bullying and cyberbullying, heavy use of online and social media utilization, ADHD and impulsivity, all of which contribute to teen suicide risk in a more powerful way than in adults.

Factors such as depression, anxiety, substance use, ADHD, learning disabilities, non-suicidal self-injury, trauma, early childhood adversity, perfectionism, and genetic loading combine with external life circumstances to push the young person toward a sense of hopelessness and feeling overwhelmed, trapped, or like a burden. And as is the case with adult suicide risk, access to lethal means plays a major part in increasing risk. An important risk factor is the presence of firearms and other lethal means in the home. Studies show that access to firearms increases suicide risk 2–5 times for youth in firearm-owning homes.[6,7] In a 2019 study of state-level firearm ownership and suicide rates, results indicated that for each 10 percentage-point increase in state-wide household firearm ownership, the state's youth suicide rate increased by 26.9%.[8]

External psychosocial stressors that increase suicide risk can include:

- family violence
- physical abuse
- sexual abuse
- rejection related to sexual orientation or gender identity
- experiences with loss or humiliation
- bullying

Adolescence Presents a Window of Opportunity To Prevent Serious Outcomes in the Short and Longer Term

Because suicidal ideation and behavior often have their first onset during adolescence, this developmental period offers an important window of opportunity to engage the youth in treatment and support which can avert a path to elevated risk of premature death, mental health, and functioning problems. Youths with suicidal ideation, attempts, and other forms of deliberate self-harm (NSSI such as cutting or burning oneself without suicidal intent) are at risk for both death by suicide and death by other unnatural causes such as alcohol and drug overdose, and accidents.[10]

Nonsuicidal Self-Injury

Nonsuicidal self-injurious behaviors are common among youth with a lifetime prevalence of 18% worldwide and include cutting, scratching, burning, and head banging. NSSI is by definition not intended to end one's life, but there are different ways of understanding NSSI. Because it has some different associated features from suicidal behavior such as positive affect and being used as a way to cope and even avoid suicide, it can be viewed as quite separate from suicidal thoughts and behaviors. However, NSSI can also be viewed as a precursor to suicidal behavior in some individuals since the presence or history of NSSI does demonstrate a higher likelihood of later developing suicidal behavior and risk of suicide. NSSI is most likely to lead to future suicidal behavior when there is a family history of suicide attempts or death, aggression, and higher levels of severity and chronicity of depression. Treatment should consider the broader clinical picture but can also target NSSI. Treatments that have been studied include DBT, CBT, mentalization therapy, and parent/family therapy. Elements across therapeutic modalities that are most effective for reducing NSSI behaviors include:

- Incorporating coping skills or safety planning
- Addressing negative affect
- Emotion regulation
- Distress tolerance
- Interpersonal skills building
- Increasing social connection and support

E Treatment of Child and Adolescent Mental Health Conditions

One in four Americans will have a mental health condition in their lifetime and 50% of these conditions have their onset by age 14; 75% by age 24. Therefore, the need to identify and treat mental health deterioration and illness in children and adolescents is compelling, and yet less than half of young people with depression and other psychiatric disorders receive treatment.

As discussed in Chapter 9 special consideration that occurred in the early 2000s was the UK's MHRA and USA's FDA decision to place warnings on all antidepressants for youth and young adult patients. In the USA the black box warning was issued for antidepressant use in patients under 24 years old for "increased risk of suicidal thinking, feeling and behavior." After this occurred, there was a documented decrease in diagnosing and treating depression in primary care during the years following the black box warning in 2004. In a large cohort study that included 1.1 million adolescents, 1.4 million young adults, and 5 million older adults, data related to mental health over a 10-year period from 2000 to 2010 was collected.[11] The study revealed significant reductions in antidepressant use within two years of the FDA advisory release: relative reductions of 31.0%, 24.3%, and 14.5% among adolescents, young adults, and older adults respectively. Even though the warning was for youth and young adults under the age of 24, the effect seemed to spill over into the identification and treatment of depression across all ages. Moreover, the use of non-pharmacologic treatments for depression and anxiety such as CBT did not increase to replace the decreases in treatment with medications.[12] This was thought to be associated with fear and confusion regarding use of antidepressants among clinical providers, as well as among parents and the general population, leading to reluctance among healthcare practitioners to appropriately treat depression with antidepressant medication.

The FDA's decision to place the black box warning on antidepressant labeling for use in young people under 24 years old was based on higher rates (4%) of suicidal ideation than placebo (2%), however, the methodology did not allow for examination of potential positive effects on suicide risk, nor incorporation of pre-study levels of suicidal ideation or behaviors.[13] Notably there were no suicide deaths and extremely few attempts in the data set on which the FDA based its decision. (See Chapter 9 for more information on the USA's FDA and UK's MHRA antidepressant warnings.)

According to the American Academy of Pediatrics, the benefits of antidepressants outweigh the potential risks to most young patients. Many studies support this opinion.[14,15] For example, one research team conducted a reanalysis of all the trials related to two medications, fluoxetine and venlafaxine.[16] The researchers did not find any evidence of increased suicidal ideation or behavior. It did find a significant significantly positive impact on depression for all age groups, but especially for youth. A total of 46.6% of young patients treated with fluoxetine witnessed a decrease in their depression compared with 16.5% of young patients treated with the placebo.[17]

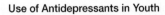

Use of Antidepressants in Youth

According to the American Academy of Pediatrics, the benefits of antidepressants outweigh the potential risks to most young patients. Many studies support this opinion.[14,15] A landmark review by child psychiatry expert Dr. John Walkup finds much of the controversy surrounding the efficacy of antidepressants for the treatment of depression in children and adolescents is related to methodological and implementation problems with industry-sponsored depression trials in children.[18] He makes a strong case for the appropriate use and efficacy of antidepressants demonstrated by National Institute of Mental Health (NIMH)-sponsored trials which, by contrast to industry trials, have many methodological strengths, lower placebo response rates (30–35%), and meaningful between-group differences that support antidepressant efficacy. This rationale combined with the clear efficacy of SSRIs for childhood onset OCD and other anxiety disorders, means there is an appropriate use of medications to address childhood/adolescent mental health conditions. See Chapter 9 for clinical guidance about use of medications in patients who may have increased risk.

Therefore it is critically important both in pediatric primary care as well as in behavioral health settings that children and adolescents be screened for changes in mental health. When suicide risk presents as a possibility, it is imperative to consider not only the child's short-term safety, but also ways to address the child's longer term mental health prognosis. Treatment for mental health problems in the child and teen years can include talk therapy (individual, group and/or family therapy) and medications, as well as higher levels of care such as intensive outpatient programs or inpatient or residential treatment. While covering all of the types of treatment for child and adolescent psychiatric conditions is outside the scope here, it is important to be aware of the psychosocial talk therapy modalities that have a growing evidence base for reducing suicide risk (shown in the text box below), and to consider which ones are available in your community or which ones you could become trained in. For any child or teen who presents with more persistent or recurrent suicidal thoughts or for youth with other suicide risk factors, not only is an evaluation for an emerging mental health condition imperative, but therapy should be strongly considered and discussed with the patient and parent.

13

Psychosocial Treatment Modalities with Evidence for Reducing Suicide Risk and Alleviating Distress

- SAFETY, a DBT-informed cognitive-behavioral treatment with a strong family focus was associated with reduced risk of suicide attempts (SAs) both at post-treatment (three months) and through 6- to 12-months of follow-up.

- Youth-Nominated Support Team Intervention for Suicidal Adolescents: Version II (YST) is associated with reduced mortality (from suicide, drug overdose, undetermined/accidental, homicide, and medical causes) 11 to 14 years after psychiatric hospitalization for suicide risk.[10]

- Integrated Cognitive Behavioral Therapy (CBT) for suicide risk and substance abuse was found to be associated with fewer SAs and improvement in substance abuse.

- Mentalization-based treatment was associated with reduced self-harm levels.

- CBT for Suicide Prevention (CBT-SP) combined with antidepressant medication in the Treatment of Adolescent Suicide Attempters (TASA) study of 12–18 year-old youth with depression and recent suicide attempt, was found to effectively treat depression and may have reduced risk of suicidal behavior especially after 12 weeks of treatment when depressive symptoms have improved.[19]

- Lethal Means Counseling: Consideration of interventions for reducing suicide risk must always include the brief intervention of counseling the patient and parents about the importance of storing all forms of lethal means outside the home if at all possible, and if not, securing them at least until the period of risk is resolved.

 Role of Social Media

Research on the effects of social media and online activities on youth mental health is emerging, complex, and shows mixed findings. On the one hand, social media and online sites can provide a source of connection and encouragement related to mental health topics for many people. However many studies' findings indicate negative trends related to mental health, for example in the case of heavy use >2–5 hours screen time per day, and bedtime use which may contribute to disruptions in sleep, depressed mood, and anxiety. Suicide risk in vulnerable teens may be impacted by social media use for the above reasons as well as the potential for cyber bullying, according to many child experts including Dr. Benjamin Shain who led the American Academy of Pediatrics Committee on Adolescence guidelines for addressing suicide risk.[20]

Internet use can also contribute to the risk of suicide contagion following a peer or celebrity suicide death or attempt. Additionally, there are publicly accessible pro-suicide websites (not only on the dark web), which encourage suicide and provide specific methods for suicide. Advocacy efforts to have these sites squelched have proven challenging to date.

The data on the relationship between social media utilization and mental health points to several mediators: nighttime use of screens is known to disrupt sleep; youth with mental health vulnerabilities may be more prone to the adverse mood and anxiety effects of social comparison, fear of missing out, and negative online interactions. Some youth may also interpret online peer interactions in more negative ways. And heavy utilization can contribute to screen or online gaming addiction.

- Guidance should include limiting screen time and for youth with mental health conditions or other vulnerabilities; this should be modified further and personalized with individual strengths and vulnerabilities in mind.
- Parents should be advised to think carefully about the age of initial provision of a smart phone for children.
- Clinicians could inquire about young patients' social media utilization since it is as "real" a part of their lives as what adults think of as "real life." Clinicians are encouraged to incorporate social media utilization into history taking and similarly utilize it as part of psychoeducation and treatment planning.

Many mental health-savvy young people are practicing a social media pause, taking breaks from social media and limiting their utilization in a number of ways (time/day, types of platforms, avoiding toxic interactions, and interacting more with positive, encouraging individuals and platforms).

G Suicide Contagion

Suicide contagion is a real phenomenon for vulnerable individuals; humans are social creatures with a hard wiring for imitation (vis-a-vis mirror neurons), and youth are more susceptible than adults likely related to their stage of psychological development and developing brain. It is estimated that for 1–5% of all teen suicides, contagion may be a relevant factor. This can occur by exposure to a peer who attempts or dies by suicide, by the way media covers a celebrity's suicide, or via the portrayal of suicide through graphic or sensationalized visual images and language in fictional and non-fiction media.[21] There is also the potential for suicide preventive impact with positive messaging in media, social media, entertainment, and music. The way media, schools, and other leaders shape messaging about a suicide death can impact the risk of contagion for vulnerable youth. An important resource for schools, parents, and community leaders is the Toolkit for Schools: After A Suicide, a guide for preventing contagion and providing postvention support created by AFSP and the Suicide Prevention Resource Center.

A suicide that is extensively covered in the media can lead to a spike in suicides, or what is known as a suicide "cluster" – when a number of suicides (usually considered three or more within a reasonably short time frame) in a particular school or community occur. While media outlets are improving in their awareness of the Safe Reporting on Suicide Media Guidelines, the internet has no such centralized controls, leading to the potential for sensationalized language that can go viral quickly.

On the other hand, the internet and social media can also be a major conduit for support. Additionally, Facebook and Instagram have initiated suicide prevention programs offering support/resources to individuals who are posting concerning messages that may indicate suicide risk. There are also many pro-social mental health campaigns such as SeizeTheAwkward that encourage education and conversation about mental health. See SeizeTheAwkward.com for tips and tutorials on how to help a struggling friend that can be shared with teen and young adult patients.

In general, when communicating with youth (or any group) about suicide, avoid providing graphic details of the method of death, avoid portraying the deceased in a glorified manner, and always provide hopeful messages and actionable ways for those in distress to get help.

 Youth Warning Signs

There are a variety of possible warning signs that may indicate increased risk of suicide. Avoid the trap of viewing concerning behavior changes in teens as normal teenage behavior.

- Talking about thinking of, wanting, or planning to die should always be considered a serious warning sign at any age, including among youth. Expressing thoughts of killing oneself should never be discounted.

- Expressing hopelessness or overwhelming emotional pain should be taken very seriously and followed up as well. Feeling trapped or like a burden to others are clear warning signs.

- Significant changes in behavior or "personality" can also be clear warning signs. Behavior changes to pay attention to include the inability to focus on school or routine tasks, and increases in substance use, becoming sad, withdrawn, tired, or apathetic or angry, agitated risk-taking, irritable, or anxious. Behavior changes include the inability to focus on school, on work, or on routine tasks. Watch also for changes in eating and sleep habits – loss of appetite or insomnia, for example.

- Low self-esteem and hopelessness about the future – feeling worthless and believing that nothing will ever change, for example – are also warning signs to pay attention to.
- A traumatic loss, which can range from the death of a loved one to a broken relationship, can present increased risk, especially if accompanied by current or recent warning signs.

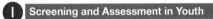

Screening and Assessment in Youth

In healthcare settings, children, teens, and young adults should be screened for changes in mental health by using instruments like the PHQ-9 depression screening instrument. It is important to note however, that the PHQ-9 is not a suicide risk screen. Data shows that a third of kids at risk for suicide are missed if they are only screened for depression. Remember that suicide risk can be driven by problems other than depression. Additionally there is no evidence that going sequentially from the PHQ-2 (if screen positive) to PHQ-9 is a valid method for suicide risk screening.[22]

For pediatric patients over the age of 10, a validated suicide screening instrument is the Ask Suicide-Screening Questions (ASQ), and the NIMH provides a toolkit for its use in pediatrics including primary care, emergency departments, and other healthcare settings.[23] The ASQ tool has been validated showing 97% sensitivity and 88% specificity for the detection of suicide risk in youth for use in primary care, emergency departments, and medical/surgical units.[24]

Youth Suicide Risk Screening Pathway

A three-tier **Suicide Risk Pathway** developed by the American Academy of Child & Adolescent Psychiatry (AACAP) was launched in 2019 by AACAP and the NIMH group under Dr. Lisa Horowitz's leadership.[25] This pathway provides guidance for screening pediatric patients for suicide risk in medical settings using the ASQ and effectively managing patients who screen positive. The three-tiered approach includes:

1. Screening for suicide risk with the ASQ (~20 seconds)
2. A brief suicide safety assessment (BSSA) to conduct a more in-depth suicide risk assessment for patients who screen positive on the ASQ ($\approx$ 10 minutes), and, if deemed necessary by the BSSA
3. A full suicide safety assessment that includes a broader mental health assessment.

To find the ASQ toolkit go to: NIMH. ASQ suicide risk screening toolkit: Screening youth for suicide risk in medical settings, www.nimh.nih.gov/ASQ

Suicide risk screening with this three-tiered approach (see "Youth Suicide Risk Screening Pathway" box) has successfully been implemented in several pediatric hospitals throughout the USA. Over 90% of 10–17-year-old patients screened for suicide risk were found to be negative with a positive identification rate of 2–4% for 10–17-year-olds and 4–11% for 10–24-year-olds.[26] This highlights both the importance of screening to identify these patients as well as the feasibility of conducting the screening without overwhelming hospital resources. By identifying key personnel who will be responsible for each tier of the screening program, and implementing a clear standardized approach to interventions at each risk level, screening can be seamlessly integrated into standards of care.

Additionally, the American Academy of Pediatrics has developed resources to equip pediatricians and families to be part of an effective safety net, such as a Youth Suicide Prevention Factsheet (Figure 13.4) that covers screening and next steps for patients who screen positive.

Recommended steps for Pediatricians

Per American Academy of Pediatrics recommendations, ask about and further assess suicide risk when indicated:

- by a positive screen for depression or any mental health concern
- by using the ASQ suicide screen
- when the patient exhibits behavioral changes at home or at school
- if the child, adolescent, or young adult speaks about feeling hopeless or overwhelmed

How to ask about suicidal ideation and other suicide risk items: It is critically important to ask the patient non-judgmentally about suicidal thoughts, ideally as part of the conversation about their life stressors and circumstances. When patients are having suicidal thoughts, and when other indicators of suicide risk are present (e.g., family reports child has been searching lethal means on the internet, having anger outbursts, expressing hopelessness, giving possessions away, etc.), it is necessary to go beyond just assessing suicidal ideation, and do a more thorough, evidence-based suicide risk assessment. For example, ask about previous periods of feeling suicidal or prior attempts; ask about how the child usually copes with conflict or stress; assess substance use; gently explore the youth's peer relationships and experiences at home. The manner in which the questions about suicide risk are presented will influence how much the child, teen, or young adult patient will open up about their experiences of distress or suicidal ideation/planning.

Figure 13.4 Youth Suicide Prevention Factsheet for Pediatricians

The American Academy of Pediatrics recommends routine screening of pediatric patients' mental health and suicide risk as indicated. When patients screen positive for suicidal ideation, this guide provides next steps consistent with other key clinical guidance, e.g., the National Action Alliance for Suicide Prevention[21] and Joint Commission Suicide Patient Safety Goal.[27] Care steps include safety planning, Lethal Means Counseling, referral, and caring follow-up communication.

Addressing Youth Suicide Prevention: A Factsheet for Primary Care Clinicians

Background:
Suicide is the 2nd leading cause of death among US youth age 15-24
Pediatricians can take important steps to protect children and families in their practice

Screening for Suicide Risk:
Choose a validated screening tool:
-Ask Suicide-Screening Questions (asQ)
-PHQ-9 Modified for Adolescents (PHQ-A)
-Columbia Suicide Severity Risk Scale (CSSRS)
Understand how to score and document results
Design a workflow for screening

Managing a Positive Screen:
Assess level of risk and intervene accordingly
-Low Risk: counsel, refer, follow-up
-Moderate Risk: counsel, refer, develop Safety Plan, follow-up
-Severe Risk: counsel, ensure parents/caregivers closely monitor child, remove lethal means, develop Safety Plan, make a crisis referral, follow-up

Counseling about Lethal Means:
Ask about access to lethal means, including firearms, medication, knives, and suffocation devices
Counsel about the importance of restricting access:
-Remove firearms from home
-Lock away medication
-Monitor belts, ropes, other suffocation devices

Ongoing Care and Follow-Up:
Help patient make a Safety Plan
-Share with parents/caregivers
-Store in EHR and send a copy home
-Templates are available
Make appropriate outpatient and/or crisis referrals
Make a "caring contact" phone call to follow-up with child and caregiver

American Academy of Pediatrics
DEDICATED TO THE HEALTH OF ALL CHILDREN*

13

The question about suicidal thoughts and plans can be embedded in the dialog, following the patient speaking of a particular stressor, and can be stated: "Does that [e.g., problem with your boyfriend] get so overwhelming that you ever think of ending your life?"

Or if asking questions as part of a screening instrument, thank the patient for sharing openly about such important matters and thank them for their honest responses. In Chapters 6–9, a full discussion of the assessment of risk and clinical care is provided.

Clinical Takeaways

- Routinely screen for mental health concerns in pediatric patients
- Screen for suicidal ideation as indicated, or routinely for age 10 and up (ASQ)
- Make time and "safe space" for patients to raise struggles/challenges they are facing
- Increase your "radar" on sensitivity for detecting distress or deterioration in mental health
- Use open, kind, non-judgmental communication and ask about suicidal thoughts
- Remember that an assessment of the patient's suicide risk does not stop with suicidal thoughts or plans. Past history, stressors, substance use, clinical course, family history, coping strategies, and support all matter to gain a broader understanding of the patient's suicide risk.
- Incorporate the topic of social media into clinical history taking and discussion with patients
- Train clinical and non-clinical staff in suicide prevention
- Incorporate safety planning and lethal means counseling into practice protocol
- Do follow-up communication with at-risk patients systematically by phone, text, cards between appointments, and especially following discharge from the emergency department or inpatient psychiatric unit
- Provide behavioral health referrals, and key crisis resources such as, in the USA, National Suicide Prevention Lifeline (1–800–273–TALK, anticipated to change to 988 in 2022) and in the USA, UK, and Ireland, Crisis Text Line (text TALK to 741741).
- Educate parents on supportive behaviors in the home for children and teens who are at risk

Clinical Care Tips

Summary recommendations for the American Academy of Pediatrics, by Dr. Joan Asarnow, a leading expert in pediatric suicide prevention:[28]

- The evaluation and management of suicide risk is feasible in pediatric care.
- This process involves four steps: **ABCD**
  - o Assess risk;
  - o Build hope and reasons for living;
  - o Connect, strengthen connections with protective adults;
  - o Develop safety plan.
- Screening tools and clinical care pathways (e.g., ASQ) have been developed to support primary care evaluation and management of suicide risk.
- Traumatic stress is associated with increased risk of suicidal behavior, underscoring the need for a trauma-informed approach.
- Every practice is different, so developing a suicide prevention approach that fits your setting is important.

13

a. Youth suicide is a global public health crisis warranting major investments, training, and action at community and clinical levels.

b. Suicide risk factors in youth include family, school, and peer interactions in addition to the universal risk factors for all ages such as unaddressed mental health conditions, lethal means availability, and genetics.

c. The clinical identification and management of emerging mental health conditions in youth is a critical aspect of youth suicide prevention.

d. Health professionals can help parents understand the behaviors in the home that protect against risk and those that increase risk.

e. Health professionals can play an important role in dispelling myths surrounding various treatment modalities in order to advocate the best treatment plan for each youth.

f. Social media plays a significant role in mental health and suicide risk for some youth. Incorporating patient experiences with social media into the clinical assessment and treatment planning is recommended.

g. Youth are more susceptible to suicide contagion than adults, therefore postvention efforts that mitigate risk after a peer or celebrity suicide are a key prevention strategy.

h. Suicide screening and assessment for youth are recommended with recently validated tools.

i. It is imperative for pediatricians, parents, school personnel, and youth workers all to play a role to prevent youth suicide.

References

1   OECD. (2017) C04.4: Teenage Suicides (15–19 Years Old). OECD Family Database. Retrieved from www.oecd.org/els/family/database.htm

2   Centers for Disease Control and Prevention. (2020) Deaths: Final Data for 2018. National Vital Statistics Report. Retrieved from www.cdc.gov/nchs/ndss/deaths.htm

3   Centers for Disease Control and Prevention. (2020) In Youth Risk Behavior Survey: Data Summary & Trends Report 2009–2019. Retrieved from www.cdc.gov/healthyyouth/data/yrbs/index.htm

4   Ruch, D. A., Sheftall, A. H., & Schlagbaum, P., et al. (2019) Trends in suicide among youth aged 10 to 19 years in the United States, 1975 to 2016. *JAMA Netw Open*, 2(5): e193886. doi: 10.1001/jamanetworkopen.2019.3886

5   Curtin, S. C. (2020) State Suicide Rates among Adolescents and Young Adults Aged 10–24: United States, 2000–2018. National Vital Statistics Reports; vol 69 no 11. Hyattsville, MD: National Center for Health Statistics.

6   Baxley, F., & Miller, M. (2006) Parental misperceptions about children and firearms. *Arch Pediatr Adolesc Med*, 160(5): 542–47.

7   Grossman, D. C., Mueller, B. A., Riedy, C., et al. (2005) Gun storage practices and risk of youth suicide and unintentional firearm injuries. *JAMA*, 293(6): 707–14. doi: 10.1001/jama.293.6.707

8   Knopov, A., Sherman, R. J., Raifman, J. R., Larson, E., & Siegel, M. B. (2019) Household gun ownership and youth suicide rates at the state level, 2005–2015. *Am J Prev Med*, 56(3): 335–42.

9   Ryan, C., Huebner, D., Diaz, R. M., & Sanchez, J. (2009) Family rejection as a predictor of negative health outcomes in white and latino lesbian, gay, and bisexual young adults. *Pediatrics*, 123(1): 346-52. doi: 10.1542/peds.2007-3524

10 King, C. A., Arango, A., Kramer, A., et al. (2019) Association of the youth-nominated support team intervention for suicidal adolescents with 11- to 14-year mortality outcomes: Secondary analysis of a randomized clinical trial. *JAMA Psychiatry*, 76(5): 492–98. doi: 10.1001/jamapsychiatry.2018.4358

11 Lu, C. Y., Zhang, F., Lakoma, M. D., et al. (2014) Changes in antidepressant use by young people and suicidal behavior after FDA warnings and media coverage: quasi-experimental study. *BMJ*, 348: g3596

12 Libby, A. M., Orton, H. D., & Valuck, R. J. (2009) Persisting decline in depression treatment after FDA warnings. *Arch Gen Psychiatry*, 66: 633–39.

13 Baldessarini, R. J., Pompili, M., & Tondo, L. (2006) Suicidal risk in antidepressant drug trials. *Arch Gen Psychiatry*, 63(3): 246–8. doi: 10.1001/archpsyc.63.3.246

14 Amy, H., Cheung, R. A., Zuckerbrot, P. S., et al. (2018) Guidelines for adolescent depression in primary care (GLAD-PC): Part II. treatment and ongoing management. *Pediatrics*, 141(3): e20174082; doi: 10.1542/peds.2017-4082

15 March, J., Silva, S., Petrycki, S., et al. (2004) Treatment for Adolescents with Depression Study (TADS) Team. Fluoxetine, cognitive-behavioral therapy, and their combination for adolescents with depression: Treatment for adolescents with depression study (TADS) randomized controlled trial. *JAMA*, 292(7): 807–20. doi: 10.1001/jama.292.7.807

16 Gibbons, R. D., Brown, C. H., Hur, K., Davis, J., & Mann, J. J. (2012) Suicidal thoughts and behavior with antidepressant treatment: Reanalysis of the randomized placebo-controlled

studies of fluoxetine and venlafaxine. *Arch Gen Psychiatry*, 69(6): 580–7. doi: 10.1001/archgenpsychiatry.2011.2048

17 Bridge, J. A., Salary, C. B., Birmaher, B., Asare, A. G., & Brent, D. A. (2005) The risks and benefits of antidepressant treatment for youth depression. *Ann Med*, 37 (6): 404–12 pmid:16203613.

18 Walkup, J. T. (2017) Antidepressant efficacy for depression in children and adolescents: industry- and NIMH-funded studies. *Am J Psychiatry*, 174(50): 430–37.

19 Vitiello, B., Brent, D. A., Greenhill, L. L., et al. (2009) Depressive symptoms and clinical status during the Treatment of Adolescent Suicide Attempters (TASA) Study. *J Am Acad Child Adolesc Psychiatry*, 48(10): 997–1004. doi: 10.1097/CHI.0b013e3181b5db66. Epub 2009 Sep 30. PMID: 20854770; PMCID: PMC2889199.

20 Shain, B., & Committee on Adolescence. (2016) Suicide and suicide attempts in adolescents. *Pediatrics*, 138(1) e20161420; doi: 10.1542/peds.2016-1420

21 The National Action Alliance for Suicide Prevention. In: National Recommendations for Depicting Suicide. Retrieved from theactionalliance.org/messaging/entertainment-messaging/national-recommendations

22 Lanzillo, E. C., Powell, D., Bridge, J. A., et al. (2017) Detecting suicide risk on pediatric inpatient medical units: Is depression screening enough? *J Am Acad Child Adolesc Psychiatry*, 56(10): S225.

23 National Institute of Mental Health. Ask Suicide-Screening Questions (ASQ) Toolkit. Retrieved from www.nimh.nih.gov/research/research-conducted-at-nimh/asq-toolkit-materials/index.shtml

24 Brahmbhatt, K., Kurtz, B. P., Afzal, K. I., et al. (2019) Suicide risk screening in pediatric hospitals: clinical pathways to address a global health crisis. *Psychosomatics*, 60(1): 1–9.

25 Horowitz, L. M. (2019) Screening for suicide risk in medical settings: Adapting research to real world implementation. *J Am Acad Child Adolesc Psychiatry*, 58(10): S320.

26 Tipton, M. V., Abernathy, T., Lanzillo, E. C., et al. (2019) Implementing suicide risk screening in pediatric primary care: From research to practice. *J Am Acad Child Adolesc Psychiatry*, 58(10).

27 Joint Commission Suicide Prevention Portal NPSG (2019). Retrieved from www.jointcommission.org/topics/suicide_prevention_portal.aspx

28 American Academy of Pediatrics. Pediatric Mental Health Minute Series: Focus on Suicide. services.aap.org/en/patient-care/mental-health-minute/suicide/. Accessed 5 November 2020.

14 Military and Veterans

Ⓐ PRINCIPLES

- Health professionals in any setting may see veterans as patients and have a key role to play in detecting risk and preventing suicide in this important, higher risk population.

- It is best to identify patients who are veterans by asking, "Have you ever served in the military?" or "Have you ever worn the uniform?"

- Cultural and experiential factors such as experiences emphasizing self-sufficiency and strength can be barriers to overcome among military and veteran patients who are experiencing distress.

- Help remind veterans and military personnel that strength includes getting help when you need it, and also remind them that we function better as a team than solo.

- Veterans in the USA die by suicide at a 1.5 increased rate compared with the civilian age-matched cohort.

- Veterans and active duty patients (and law enforcement as well) have a much higher incidence of firearm suicide than other populations. Therefore, lethal means counseling and including family members when possible is all the more critical.

- Periods of transition during military life can increase suicide risk, and therefore are important times to increase support, access to care, and screening of risk.

B Introduction

As a healthcare provider, consider taking special notice of your patients who are veterans or active duty service members. You may be the only caregiver poised to recognize suicide risk in your patients who have served. Consider always asking patients, "Have you ever served in the military?" or "Have you ever worn the uniform?" (Some veterans do not know they qualify as a veteran and therefore it may not be effective to ask, "Are you a veteran?")

Of the 17–20 US veterans who die by suicide each day, only 6 are receiving healthcare at the Veterans Health Administration (VHA). So it is up to other non-VHA clinical and community organizations to serve as a safety net that detects suicide risk and cares for veterans.

While active duty military service members and veterans are different groups, because of the overlap in experience between the groups they are being presented together in this section. Service members and veterans share similarities, notably a culture of self-reliance and potential fear of jeopardizing their career by seeking mental health services. Additionally, many veterans do not seek mental health treatment or are not forthcoming during treatment related to concerns that providers may take their firearms.

Military service experience can be viewed along a trajectory with transitions occurring at key points, including the transition when starting military training/service, pre- and post-deployment, and transitioning to civilian life into veteran status. Times of transition present challenges for all people, but particularly for those with risk factors. So as a healthcare provider to a military or veteran patient, it is important to make note of these life and career transitions and inquire about their mental health at these key times.

C Prevalence and Trends

- Since the beginning of the wars in Afghanistan and Iraq (in 2001 and 2003 respectively), the suicide rate among US veterans has risen and is now higher than general population rates.
- According to a 2019 VHA study based on 50 million veteran records from 1979 to 2017:[1]
  - An average of 17 veterans die from suicide every day.
  - In 2017, the suicide rate for veterans was 1.5 times the rate for non-veteran adults, after adjusting for population differences in age and sex.

- After adjusting for age, the rate of suicide among women veterans was 2.2 times the rate among non-veteran women.
- After adjusting for age, the rate of suicide among male veterans was 1.3 times higher than the rate among non-veteran males.

o Over 70% of male veteran suicides are by firearms and firearms accounted for 43% of female veteran suicide deaths.

o Veterans aged 18–34 had the highest suicide rate in 2017 of all age ranges (44.5 per 100,000).

o The absolute number of suicides was highest among veterans 55–74 years. This group accounted for 38% of all veteran suicides.

o Only 6 of the 17–20 veterans who take their lives each day are enrolled in the VHA. This means many at-risk veterans must be reached in healthcare and community settings outside the VHA.

Figure 14.1 and 14.2 Suicide methods in the non-veteran general population, males and females, USA (2017)

Suicide methods among US males (first pie chart) and females (second pie chart) are different with males using firearms more and females using ingestion more. Methods for suicide also vary by other demographic factors such as region, culture, and availability of particular lethal means.

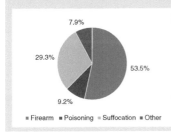

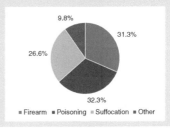

14

Key Facts

- As is true for suicide risk in general populations, suicide risk for military personnel and veterans is multifactorial.
- While deployment can destabilize individuals with baseline vulnerabilities, deployment is not thought to be a standalone cause of suicide.

Figures 14.3 and 14.4 Suicide methods among male and female US veterans

Firearms as a method among veteran suicide decedents is overrepresented among both males (first pie chart) and females (second pie chart) compared with the non-veteran population.

Source: US Department of Veteran's Affairs, Office of Mental Health and Suicide Prevention, 2019 National Veteran Suicide Prevention Annual Report

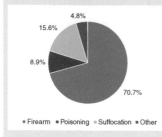

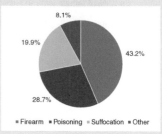

D Risk Factors

- While deployment can destabilize individuals with baseline vulnerabilities, it is not thought to be a standalone cause of suicide. In fact, some data show suicide rates are higher among service members who had not deployed compared with those who had.

- Transitions are generally times of higher suicide risk, and for military service members, this importantly includes the transition points of service members. For example, several studies have found elevated risk for soldiers within four months following the end of their deployment.[2]

- Studies show that combat experience itself is not a leading risk factor for veteran suicide. A 2013 study found that longer deployments, multiple deployments, and combat experience did **not** increase the risk for suicide among veterans.[2]

- The study, Army Study to Assess Risk and Resilience in Service members (Army STARRS) found that while suicide rates for veterans who had been deployed doubled between 2004 and 2009, suicide rates for veterans who had **never** been deployed tripled in the same period.[3]

- That said, we should not underestimate the potential impact of combat and deployment as potential risk factors for some, given that the effect of these experiences may not appear immediately. PTSD can appear gradually. And PTSD can lead to depression, alcohol, or substance abuse – all risk factors for suicide that may have their roots in the combat experience for some individuals.

- Additionally, the majority of veterans, even those who experience trauma or combat, do not develop PTSD. Many service members and veterans with a history of trauma function very well until transitions such as retirement, when there can be a sudden onset of symptoms of PTSD.

- Instead suicide risk factors for military service members and veterans more commonly include: alcohol and other substance use, psychiatric conditions – at times undiagnosed prior to entering the service – problems with work, head injury and other causes of disability, legal or financial setbacks, broken relationships, and **any period of transition** when other suicide risk factors are present. Perhaps the greatest risk factor is not the combat experience but the difficult return to civilian life.

- Mental health conditions that elevate suicide risk are very similar to general population mental health risk factors: depression, PTSD, substance use problems, psychosis, personality disorders, anxiety, and bipolar disorder. The Army STARRS study found about a third of soldiers who attempted suicide between 2004 and 2009 had mental health problems **before** they joined the Army.[3]

- Military sexual trauma is another risk factor for all veterans, but particularly among women veterans. Rates of Military Sexual Trauma (MST) are high with 20 to 45% of women veterans reporting sexual trauma while in the military.[4] Male veterans also experience MST and there is likely underreporting due to stigma for both men and women, but particularly for male victims of sexual assault.

- Another challenge is the "macho" culture of the military that creates barriers to addressing health and psychosocial needs. Cultures that celebrate strength, control, and stoicism unintentionally push people in need of help to hide their problems so as not to appear weak in front of their peers. Some major steps in meeting this challenge are being taken, with more service members and retired top commanders being willing to come forward publicly about their own struggles. In his research for the groundbreaking book, *The Invisible Front: Love and Loss in an Era of Endless War,* author Yoshi Dreazen encountered both stigma and encouraging breakthroughs in military culture.[5]

Resources for Veterans and Military Suicide Prevention

Resources for Veterans and Military Suicide Prevention

- Veterans Crisis Line 1–800–273-TALK (8255), military and veterans press 1
- Veteranscrisisline.net, call/text/chat 24/7
- BeThere Peer Support Call and Outreach Center 844–357-PEER (7337)
  Text 480–360-6188, BeTherePeerSupport.org
- Virtual Hope Box Mobile App http://t2health.dcoe.mil/apps/virtual-hope-box
- Vets 4 Warriors 855–838-8255
- Office of Warrior Care Policy, warriorcare.dodlive.mil
- InTransition, intransition.dcoe.mil
- Military One Source 1–800–342–9647, militaryonesource.mil
- Tragedy Assistance Program for Survivors (TAPS) 1–800–959–8277, taps.org
- Coaching Into Care, a resource for loved ones of veterans who are struggling, but who are reluctant to enter treatment 1–888–823–7458 or coachingintocare@va.gov

 KEY TAKEAWAYS

a. Suicide prevention for veterans must also occur robustly in health- and community-based settings outside the Veterans Health Administration since the majority of US veterans who die by suicide do not receive their healthcare from the VHA.

b. Ask patients, "Have you ever served in the military?" or "Have you ever worn the uniform?" rather than "Are you a veteran?"

c. Veterans in the US die by suicide at 1.5 times the rate of their civilian age-matched cohort.

d. Cultural factors that emphasize self-sufficiency and strength tend to be barriers to seeking support or mental health treatment among military and veteran patients who are experiencing distress.

e. Remind veterans and military personnel that staying strong requires getting help when you need it, and also remind them that we function better as a team than solo. There is no weakness in getting support and treatment.

f. Veterans and active duty patients have a much higher incidence of firearm suicide than other populations. Therefore, lethal means counseling and communication with family members when possible about making the home environment safe especially during periods of higher risk are critical.

g. Periods of transition in military personnel lives are important times to increase support, access to care, and screen for increased risk.

14

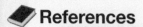

References

1   **US Department of Veterans Affairs. (2019)** 2019 National Veteran Suicide Prevention Annual Report. Retrieved from www.mentalhealth.va.gov/docs/data-sheets/2019/2019_National_Veteran_Suicide_Prevention_Annual_Report_508.pdf

2   **LeardMann, C. A., Powell, T. M., Smith, T. C., et al. (2013)** Risk factors associated with suicide in current and former US Military personnel. *JAMA*, 310(5): 496–506. doi: 10.1001/jama.2013.65164

3   **Naifeh, J. A., Herberman Mash, H. B., Stein, M. B., et al. (2019)** The Army Study to Assess Risk and Resilience in Service members (Army STARRS): Progress toward understanding suicide among soldiers. *Mol Psychiatry*, 24: 34–48. doi: 10.1038/s41380-018-0197-z

4   **Suris, A., & Lind, L. (2008)** Military sexual trauma: A review of prevalence and associated health trauma in veterans. *Trauma, Violence & Abuse*, 9: 250–69.

5   **Dreazen, Y. (2015)** *The Invisible Front: Love and Loss in an Era of Endless War*. New York: Penguin Random House.

15

Older Adults

A Introduction

Although suicide in other demographic groups may receive more public attention, suicide among older adults has long been an intense target of concern for suicide prevention. In fact, in most populations and regions of the world, suicide rates are highest in older or middle age adults. Older adult suicide is also an area where the suicide prevention field has learned a lot about successful prevention programs that utilize a combination of clinical and social/community programs.

B PRINCIPLES

a. Older adult suicide is a longstanding public health crisis.

b. Suicide rates in older age adults are often the highest of any age group, especially among developed nations.

c. Older adult suicide is complex with converging risk factors including unaddressed mental health conditions, disability from both mental and physical health problems, social isolation, losses of peers, autonomy, and sense of identity, youth-idolizing culture that devalues older age members of families and society, economic changes, and even potential cohort effects in some instances.

245

d. It is important for clinicians to guard against erroneous "common sense" assumptions, for example, if I were in their shoes (e.g., loss of autonomy or chronic pain) I'd also be depressed or suicidal. Clinical depression and suicide risk are not normal responses at any age.

e. It is critically important to identify and address the most potent risk factors for suicide among older adults, "The 4 D's": Depression, Disease/Disability, Disconnectedness, and Deadly means.

f. A multi-prong suicide prevention strategy for older adults includes community, family, policy, and clinical interventions.

 Scope of the Problem and Trends

In most parts of the world, older adults have the highest rates of suicide. Suicide in both middle and later life are critical targets for prevention, given the highest rates in almost all countries occur among middle or older adults. Although suicide attempts are more frequent among adolescents and young adults, middle and older age men and women show the highest suicide rates in most developed countries.[1,2] In contrast, in many low- and middle-income countries, suicide rates peak in young adulthood.[3]

 Figure 15.1 Suicides globally by age, showing high and low country-level income

In most high-income nations, middle and older age adults have the highest suicide rates. In low- and middle-income countries, suicide rates peak in young adulthood.[2]

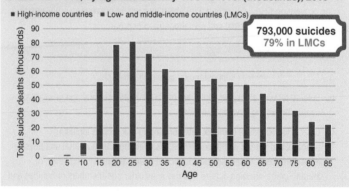

Older adults have historically had the highest rates of suicide in developed nations, including in the UK, USA, Australia, Denmark, and other European countries. However, middle age suicide rates are also notably high and in Canada and the USA have surpassed older demographic age groups. Older Canadian and American adults' rates remain high however, and the lethality of attempt behavior rises over the course of the life cycle. In the older years, attempts tend to be more lethal with the attempt to death ratio approximately 4:1 (versus in youth where the attempts to death ratio is approximately 100:1).[1]

In other countries, the relationship of aging with suicide risk varies. In China older adults' suicide rates have increased in recent years even while the overall national suicide rate has declined; the past three decades have witnessed a remarkable drop in overall suicide rates in China from 17.6 per 100,000 in 1987 to 7.46 in 2014. This decline is thought to be driven by sharp decreases in the rate of younger Chinese people during recent years of urbanization and new opportunities, while older Chinese rates continue to rise.[4]

A number of factors influence suicide risk among middle and older age adults, including physical and mental health-related disability, stressors common to this life stage, economic trends, societal views and roles of older adults, unmet expectations, isolation, and losses.

Cohort effects may also play a role. In the USA, throughout their entire life cycle over many decades, the Baby Boomer generation (born 1946–1964) has had higher suicide rates (and other psychosocial problems) than any other previous generation. As Boomers make up an increasingly large part of the older population, this means that the rate among older Americans could unfortunately rise if this cohort effect continues.[5]

The suicide method for older adults varies around the world. In the USA, older adults have significantly higher rates of firearm suicide than younger Americans, highlighting the rate of fatality of attempts by older adults generally being much higher than for younger populations.[6]

In older age Americans, the gender gap widens especially for older White men, whose rates are 6 to 8 times higher than older age White women. For African American men, suicide rates peak in the young adult years. African American females are the demographic group with the lowest rates of suicide in the USA.

15

Figure 15.2 Suicide rates by age, with gender and race, in the USA

Suicide rates tend to be higher among older adults, although in some groups such as Black males and both Black and White females in the USA, rates are lower in older adults.

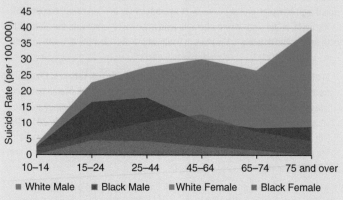

Source: CDC, National Vital Statistics Reports, Deaths: Final Data for 2017

D **Risk Factors for Older Age Adults: The 4 D's**

The 4 D's of Suicide Risk in Older Age

The 4 D's is a summary of the main suicide risk factors for older adults by Dr. Yeates Conwell, a leading expert in older adult suicide prevention.[7,8]

1. Depression
2. Disease/Disability
3. Disconnectedness
4. Deadly means

Recommendations for Addressing the 4 D's

1. Aggressively screen and treat depression in older adults.

2. Address the concerns of patients concerning their illnesses including the illnesses' psychological impacts on autonomy, identity, suffering, and anxiety. Optimize patients' functioning to every extent possible in order to minimize the disabling impact of illnesses. Treating depression and anxiety is critical to this when they are present.

3. Involve family and "prescribe" various social activities and services.

4. Counsel patients on lethal means. Ensure any lethal methods including firearms, dangerous medications, and substances, are secured or stored outside the patient's home. Involve family in this discussion when possible.[7-9]

● "Depression": Mental Health, Suicide Attempts, and Treatment

- Older people with mental health conditions are even less likely to receive treatment for their psychiatric condition than young adults. They do access healthcare through primary care, which means that in many cases of an older adult who is at risk for suicide, the only healthcare professional who may have an opportunity to detect risk is in primary care.

- Several studies have shown that up to a half of the older adults who died by suicide had seen their primary care provider in the week prior – and three quarters of them had seen their doctor in the last month of their lives.[10]

- Although a third of older adults who died by suicide had seen a mental health provider at some earlier point, very few were in treatment at the time of suicide.[11]

- Studies, including a 2014 Danish study, have shown that patients over 50 who were prescribed antidepressants were less likely to attempt suicide. Aggressive treatment of depression and other mental health conditions can have a significant impact in reducing suicides in this age group.[12]

- Psychological autopsy studies reveal that the majority (85% to 100%) of older adult suicides have a psychiatric condition which contributes to their death by suicide.[13]

- Older age suicide decedents are 50 to 60 times more likely to suffer from major depression than the general population of older adults.[2]

15

- Several studies involving both older and younger patients have linked cognitive dysfunction, specifically frontal executive function, to suicidal ideation and attempts.[1]
- Further studies indicate that vascular disease may also be a contributing factor to late onset depression and suicidal ideation and attempts.
- Older adults who attempted suicide in the past are significantly more likely to attempt suicide again. As is true across the lifespan, a history of suicide attempts is a very significant risk factor for this age group.[1]

● Disease and Disability

- Physical illness is a risk factor for suicide, but given the large majority of older patients who have several medical conditions, this risk factor alone may not be as helpful in detecting suicide risk. Honing in on specific concerns – pain or disability which are known to increase suicide risk – is highly recommended. **Addressing pain and decreasing the disabling impact of illness can reduce the likelihood of suicide.**
- Another key factor to look for in older adults is depression as a standalone concern or comorbid or secondary to physical health conditions. Depression is **not** a natural part of aging, and while pain and disability make depression more likely, it does not mean depression will not have serious negative effects of its own. **Depression is a key target for screening and treatment among older adults.**
- One illness on its own does not usually lead to suicide, but older people – as opposed to younger people – often suffer from a variety of acute and chronic physical problems. This accumulation can be overwhelming psychologically, and can also exert direct physiological effects on the brain and body.
- Several studies have found a correlation between chronic pain and suicide.[14]

● Disconnectedness

- **There is a high correlation between suicide and social disconnectedness**. The following factors have been strongly associated with protecting against suicide risk: the presence of one confidante, living with peers/family versus alone, being active in community activities, with an organization or with a hobby, and the decreased likelihood of suicide. Older people who feel lonely, experience a high degree of interpersonal discord, or feel that they are a burden to those around them have much higher risk of suicide.[1,2]

- A meta-analysis of 148 studies on the relationship between social connections and overall general mortality finds a 50% increased likelihood of survival for people with stronger social relationships. Furthermore, they note the influence of social disconnectedness on risk for death is comparable to or greater than that associated with well-established risk factors such as smoking, obesity, and physical inactivity.[15]
- Thus, a strong support network of family, friends, peers, or social support services are of critical importance in preventing suicide.
- Studies of post-discharge contact alone demonstrate that various forms of communication with high risk patients several times in the following year reduces suicide risk.[16]
- Family discord is also a known risk factor for suicide among older people.[17]

● Deadly Means

- The lethality of suicide-attempt behavior increases over the life cycle. In the teen years, the attempt:death ratio is estimated to be as much as 100–200:1, whereas in older age adults, the ratio is estimated as 4:1.[18]
- The reasons for the high lethality among older adults' attempts are thought to relate to:
    - ○ Older adults may plan more carefully and use more deadly methods.
    - ○ Older adults are less likely to be discovered and rescued.
    - ○ The generally greater physical frailty of older adults means they may be less likely to recover from an attempt.
- For any older age patient at risk of suicide, it is therefore imperative to consider the lethal means accessible to them in their home and general environment. Counseling on firearms and other lethal means is an extremely important part of the clinical care for older adults who are at risk.

● Suicide Prevention Strategies

A combination of community and clinical interventions can prevent suicide among older people. As or more critical than with other populations, a multi-prong approach that includes community resources, social support, and clinical treatment that address both mental health conditions as well as physical medical illness and disability are critical to preventing suicide among older adults.

KEY TAKEAWAYS

a. Older adult suicide is a longstanding public health crisis.

b. Suicide rates among older age adults are often the highest of any age group, especially among developed nations.

c. It is critically important to identify and address the 4 D's – the most potent risk factors for suicide among older adults: Depression, Disease/Disability, Disconnectedness, and Deadly means.

d. A multi-prong suicide prevention strategy for older adults includes community, family, policy, and clinical interventions.

Clinical Takeaways in the Care of Older Patients

- Detect and aggressively treat depression and anxiety.

- Work with family members and community resources to maximize social connectedness and activity level.

- "Prescribe" activities that enhance social connections with peers and/or family members or activities such as volunteering and exploring service opportunities.

- Minimize the level of disability associated with medical and psychiatric illnesses.

- Make every effort to make the patient's environment safe. Provide lethal means counseling and involve family and caregivers to help ensure that firearms and toxic substances and medications are secured or stored off-site.

References

1   Conwell, Y., & Thompson, C. (2008). Suicidal behavior in elders. *Psychiatr Clin North Am*, 31(2): 333–56.

2   Conwell, Y., Van Orden, K., & Caine, E. D. (2011) Suicide in older adults. *The Psychiatric Clinics of North America*, 34(2): 451–ix. doi: 10.1016/j.psc.2011.02.002

3   World Health Organization. (2019) Suicide Prevention. Retrieved from www.who.int/mental_health/suicide-prevention/age_income_level_2016.JPG?ua=1

4   Zhong, B. L., Chiu, H. F. K., & Conwell, Y. (2016) Elderly suicide trends in the context of transforming China, 1987–2014. *Sci Rep*, 6. Retrieved from www.nature.com/articles/srep37724

5   Phillips, J. A. (2013). Factors associated with temporal and spatial patterns in suicide rates across U.S. states, 1976–2000. *Demography*, 50(2): 591–614.

6   Conwell, Y., Duberstein, P. R., Cox, C., et al. (1998) Age differences in behaviors leading to completed suicide. *Am J Geriatr Psychiatry*, 6(2): 122–26.

7   Conwell, Y. (2014) Suicide later in life: Challenges and priorities for prevention. *Am J Prev Med*, 47(3): Supplement 2, S244–S250.

8   American Foundation for Suicide Prevention. The Four D's of Suicide Risk in Older Adults with Dr. Yeates Conwell. Retrieved from afsp.org/our-work/research/meet-the-researchers-an-introduction-to-the-latest-in-suicide-research/

9   Lapierre, S., Erlangsen, A., Waern, M., De Leo, D., Oyama, H., Scocco, P., et al. (2011) A systematic review of elderly suicide prevention programs. *Crisis*, 32(2), 88–98. doi: 10.1027/0227-5910/a000076

10   Luoma, J. B., Martin, C. E., & Peason, J. L. (2002) Contact with mental health and primary care providers before suicide: A review of the evidence. *Am J Psychiatry*, 159(6): 909–16.

11   Ahmedani, B. K., Simon, G. E., Stewart, C., et al. (2014) Health care contacts in the year before suicide death. *J Gen Intern Med*, 29: 870.

12   Erlangsen, A., & Conwell, Y. (2014) Age-related response to redeemed antidepressants measured by completed suicide in older adults: a nationwide cohort study. *Am J Geriatr Psychiatry*, 22(1): 25–33. doi: 10.1016/j.jagp.2012.08.008

13   Cavanagh, J. T., Carson, A. J., Sharpe, M., & Lawrie, S .M. (2003) Psychological autopsy studies of suicide: A systematic review. *Psychol Med*, 33(3): 395–405.

14   Hooley, J. M., Franklin, J. C., & Nock, M. K. (2014) Chronic pain and suicide: Understanding the association. *Curr Pain Headache Rep*, 18: 435.

15   Holt-Lunstad, J., Smith, T. B., & Layton, J. B. (2010) Social relationships and mortality risk: A meta-analytic review. *PLoS Med*, 7(7): e1000316.

16   Luxton, D. D., June, J. D., & Comtois, K. A. (2013) Can postdischarge follow-up contacts prevent suicide and suicidal behavior? A review of the evidence. *Crisis*, 34(1): 32–41.

17   Duberstein, P. R., Conwell, Y., Conner, K. R., et al. (2004) Suicide at 50 years of age and older: Perceived physical illness, family discord and financial strain. *Psychol Med*, 34(1): 137–46.

18   McIntosh, J. L., Santos, J. F., Hubbard, R. W., & Overholser, J. C. (1994) *Elder Suicide: Research, Theory, and Treatment.* Washington, DC: American Psychological Association.

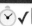

16

LGBTQ Populations

 QUICK CHECK

Ⓐ Introduction: Stigma and Risk

- In recent years in the USA, UK, and many other areas around the world, awareness of suicide risk in LGBTQ youth as well as across the lifespan has increased considerably. While these advances are critically important, stigma reduction occurs at different paces, unevenly around the world, and, even within small communities, widely varying attitudes exist. Therefore, while progress has been profound in many places, there is much work still to be done to eradicate discrimination and stigma.

- An estimated 4.5% of the population is LGBTQ, likely an underestimate.[2]

- Research shows that lesbian and gay people have several times greater rates of suicidal ideation and attempts compared with heterosexual populations.[2]

- For bisexual and transgender (trans) people, rates of ideation and attempts are even greater. For example, several studies show gay and bisexual males are four times more likely to attempt suicide than heterosexual males, while lesbian and bisexual females are twice as likely to attempt suicide.[3,4]

- The transgender population is perhaps the most at-risk population, with more than 40% of trans adults attempting suicide at one point in their lives (compared to less than 5% for the general population).[5] More specific information on trans suicide risk factors and related issues is provided below.

- Because the US Standard Certificate of Death does not include sexual orientation or gender identity (SOGI), there is not currently systematic surveillance for rate or number of suicide deaths among lesbian, gay, bisexual, or transgender (LGBT) people anywhere in the world, although some US states' surveillance is in the early stages of implementation to systematically include SOGI as part of the vital statistics death record. This has been an advocacy and education effort at AFSP and the Johnson Family Foundation.[6]

B PRINCIPLES

- While culture in many regions is changing, stigma, discrimination, family rejection, bullying, and abuse unfortunately continue to be common experiences among LGBTQ people, leading to increased suicide risk in this population. (Please see more detailed examples of behaviors in the home that impact outcomes for LGBTQ youth based on research by the Family Acceptance Project in Chapter 13 on Youth, p. 221.)

- Among LGBTQ people, trans people are likely to have the highest risk for suicide, but gay, lesbian, and bisexual people also have elevated rates of suicidal behavior.

- Clinicians can counsel and support LGBTQ patients, provide opportunities to address mental health conditions, and screen for suicidal ideation or past behavior to process prior trauma and to discuss their current concerns. All of these actions accrue toward reducing suicide risk.

- Clinicians should counsel parents and families about the recommendations on behavior in the home and the need to provide acceptance and support for their LGBTQ loved one, and this behavioral choice does not need to be reliant on changing their own personal value system.

- Clinicians should have a low threshold for providing psychological support and behavioral healthcare referral since the risk-producing effects of discrimination and trauma can be mitigated powerfully through therapy, support, and processing.

16

Clinicians can counsel and support LGBTQ patients, provide opportunities to address mental health conditions, and screen for suicidal ideation or past behavior to process prior trauma and to discuss their current concerns. All of these actions accrue toward reducing suicide risk.

LGBTQ Risk and Protective Factors

- The risk factors for LGBTQ people are similar for general populations but with notable differences in rates of discrimination and other forms of duress.
- Risk factors include mental health problems, depression, anxiety disorders, and substance abuse. The high rates of stigma and discrimination LGBTQ people suffer are known to increase the likelihood of mental health problems and suicide risk. Perhaps one of the greatest contributors to the deterioration of mental health in LGBTQ people, especially youth, is the experience of being rejected by family.[7]
- Research findings demonstrate that LGBTQ youth are three times more likely to attempt suicide than their heterosexual and cisgender peers.
- Support and acceptance by the family is a strongly protective factor for LGBTQ youth.[8] The support of caring adults outside the family and a positive self identity can also contribute to the protection of LGBTQ youth. For more information about the critical importance of family support for LGBTQ youth, please see Family Acceptance Project research, posters, and other resources.[9]

 More Information about Transgender People and Risk

- As noted earlier, the transgender population is one of the most at-risk populations, with a 41% lifetime risk of attempting suicide (compared to 4.6% for the general population).[10]
- As with gay, lesbian, and bisexual people, family rejection is a major risk factor for trans people. One study showed that 57% of trans people who had been rejected by their families had attempted suicide.[10]
- Another important risk factor is violence or physical or sexual abuse as a result of transgender identity. The more frequent or intense the abuse, according to studies, the more likely the trans person is to attempt suicide.[11]
- The figures for harassment and violence are stark. Studies find:
  o 50% of trans people who had been harassed or bullied at school had attempted suicide.
  o 55% of trans people who had been discriminated against or harassed at work had attempted suicide.
  o 65% of trans people who had suffered sexual violence at work and 70% who had suffered sexual violence at school had attempted suicide.[10]

Sensitive Discussions about Disclosing or Transitioning

The issue of disclosure and transition is a complicated one. Those whose trans identity is visible – or those who disclose identity – may experience greater discrimination, physical abuse, and harassment, leading to potentially greater risk compared with those whose gender identity is less visible. This is balanced by the risk of not being out or transitioned, which includes the significant psychological burden of keeping parts of one's identity compartmentalized, and having to keep secrets.

Even though you as a health professional may have strong advocacy feelings and views about LGBTQ people, and although culture is changing in many regions of the world, until stigma is eradicated, counseling on the question of whether to disclose or transition should be highly customized to the individual, making them aware of the potential risks and benefits that can come with disclosure or transitioning.

- Psychological ambivalence related to how a trans individual feels about their own identify can create additional burden. Providing or referring for expert therapy to discuss these types of issues can be extremely helpful.

- Known general risk factors – such as substance abuse, depression, homelessness – are often present and unfortunately more commonly experienced among transgender people.

- Further complicating the challenges trans people face is the fact that, as a review of several studies indicates, transgender people may be less likely than the general population to seek professional help for mental health struggles.[3,11]

Clinical Tips

- Remember that most LGBTQ patients will have already had experiences of rejection, bullying, trauma, or assault, and therefore safety and trust in the clinical relationship is important to establish.

- Ensure that communication with LGBTQ patients is prefaced and interspersed with clear statements of support and empathy to optimize open dialog and patients' perception of "safety" in the therapeutic relationship.

- Express support for patients' challenging experiences so that at-risk patients feel a sense of being understood, heard, and supported, which is a critical part of their safety net. This is true in primary care, as well as specialty care including behavioral health.

- Remember that referring to therapy or behavioral health does not need to be reserved for crisis or severe mental health conditions.

16

Clinical Takeaways

- It is critically important for patients who are gay, bisexual, or trans to have the opportunity to receive supportive and appropriate medical care, and to process the experiences such as previous family or peer rejection and bullying or abuse at school or at work. The opportunity to process and work through experiences of discrimination and family rejection – current or past – can lead to more positive outcomes related to suicide risk.

- It is also important to give LGBTQ patients the opportunity to discuss their perceptions of their sexual identity, and their sense of confidence or ambivalence related to issues of identity.

- It is important to realize that in the current reality and cultural values of most societies around the world, even in areas where more progress related to LGBTQ acceptance has occurred, the experience of coming out or transitioning remains complicated for many. Therefore, transgender transition is a very individual decision that warrants professional, specialized mental health support and medical consultation, to consider the question of if and when to approach gender transition.

- All patients including LGBTQ patients should be referred to a mental health professional for therapy or psychiatric treatment when it can be helpful. In other words, behavioral health referral does not need to be reserved for crisis or severe mental health conditions.

- There is strong evidence that particular behaviors in the home (rejecting behaviors and words) increase suicide risk for LGBTQ youth, and conversely that supportive behaviors in the home can reduce risk.[7,8,12]

- Even when lower level distress is present, which may indicate subsyndromal symptoms of MDD, anxiety, or PTSD, treatment can be critically helpful for short- and long-term outcomes and can even potentially prevent later worsening or crisis. Mental health professionals can help patients process the intense and cumulative life challenges present for many LGBTQ people in a socially rejecting culture.

- Remember to pay attention to all other risk factors such as personal and family mental health history and prior suicidal behavior, in addition to trauma and adverse experiences related and unrelated to LGBTQ status.

KEY TAKEAWAYS

a. While the prevailing culture in many regions is changing toward greater understanding about sexual orientation and gender identity, stigma, discrimination, family rejection, bullying, and abuse unfortunately continue to be common experiences among LGBTQ people, leading to increased suicide risk in this population.

b. There are many actions clinicians can take that reduce suicide risk in LGBTQ patients. Clinicians can counsel and support LGBTQ patients, provide opportunities to address mental health conditions, screen for suicidal ideation or past behavior, process prior trauma, and discuss their current concerns. All of these actions accrue toward reducing suicide risk.

c. Clinicians should counsel parents and families about the recommendations on behavior in the home, and the need to provide love and support for their LGBTQ family member, which does not require them to change their value system.

d. Have a low threshold for providing psychological support and behavioral healthcare referral since the risk-producing effects of discrimination and trauma can be mitigated powerfully through therapy, support, and processing.

16

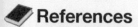

References

1 UCLA Williams Institute. williamsinstitute.law.ucla.edu/visualization/lgbt-stats/?topic= LGBT#density. Accessed February 29, 2020.

2 Movement Advancement Project. (2017) In: Talking about Suicide & LGBT Populations. Retrieved from afsp.org/wp-content/uploads/2016/01/talking-about-suicide-and-lgbt-populations-2nd-edition.pdf

3 Movement Advancement Project. (2016) Invisible Majority: The Disparities Facing Bisexual People and How to Remedy Them. Retrieved from www.lgbtmap.org/policy-and-issue-analysis/invisible-majority

4 Blosnich, J., Farmer, G. W., Lee, J. G., et al. (2014) Health inequalities among sexual minority adults: Evidence from ten U.S. states. *American Journal of Preventive Medicine*, 46(4): 337–49, doi: 10.1016/j. amepre.2013.11.010

5 Goldblum, P., Testa, R. J., Hendricks, M. L., Bradford, J., & Bongar, B. (2012) The relationship between gender-based victimization and suicide attempts in transgender people. *Professional Psychology: Research and Practice*, 43: 468–75, doi: 10.1037/a0029605

6 Haas, A. P., Lane, A., & Working Group for Postmortem Identification of SO/GI (2015) Collecting sexual orientation and gender identity data in suicide and other violent deaths: A step towards identifying and addressing LGBT mortality disparities. *LGBT Health*, 2(1): 84–87. doi: 10.1089/lgbt.2014.0083

7 Ryan, C., Huebner, D., Diaz, R. M., & Sanchez, J. (2009) Family rejection as a predictor of negative health outcomes in white and Latino lesbian, gay and bisexual young adults. *Pediatrics*, 123(1): 346–52.

8 Ryan, C., Russell, S. T., Huebner, D., Diaz, R., & Sanchez, J. (2010) Family acceptance in adolescence and the health of LGBT young adults. *Journal of Child and Adolescent Psychiatric Nursing*, 23: 205–13.

9 Family Acceptance Project. (2019) New Research-Based Poster Series Launched to Build Healthy Futures for LGBTQ & Gender Diverse Children & Youth. Retrieved from familyproject.sfsu.edu/news-announce/healthy-futures-poster-series

10 Haas, A. P., Rodgers, P. L., & Herman, J. L. (2014) Suicide Attempts among Transgender and Gender Non-Conforming Adults. American Foundation for Suicide Prevention & The Williams Institute. Retrieved from williamsinstitute.law.ucla.edu/wp-content/uploads/AFSP-Williams-Suicide-Report-Final.pdf

11 Grant, J. M., Mottet, L. A., Tanis, J., Harrison, J., Herman, J. L., & Keisling, M. (2011) Injustice at Every Turn: A Report of the National Transgender Discrimination Survey. Washington: National Center for Transgender Equality and National Gay and Lesbian Task Force. www .thetaskforce.org/static_html/downloads/reports/reports/ntds_full.pdf

12 Family Acceptance Project – Caitlin Ryan, PhD. familyproject.sfsu.edu/poster. Accessed February 29, 2020.

17 Suicide Loss Survivors

Grief is the form love takes when someone we love dies.[1]

M. Katherine Shear, M.D.

Ⓐ PRINCIPLES

- Suicide loss produces a profoundly impactful experience, which can be traumatizing for many.

- It is helpful for clinicians across specialty areas to appreciate the complexities in order to provide optimal patient care to patients who have experienced suicide loss.

- The loved one who died by suicide and their memory can be integrated into one's life moving forward, but people do not "get over" the loss of a loved one.

- Suicide loss has several known associated health outcomes affecting both physical and mental health, as well as increasing suicide risk for some.

261

- Clinicians should monitor for the potential development of Complicated Grief (CG) or Prolonged Grief Disorder, which occurs in a high percentage of people bereaved by suicide. Evidence-based treatment for CG is Complicated Grief Therapy (CGT).

- Other health sequelae of suicide loss (physical and mental health changes) should be vigilantly screened for and addressed.

- Clinicians can also experience significant personal and professional ramifications of losing a patient to suicide and recommendations are provided.

Key Point

Patients who are bereaved by suicide benefit from the care of clinicians who are knowledgeable about the intensity of the grief experience, the complex and uneven course of emotions, and the fairly common clinical sequelae that can be addressed.

B Introduction

Grief is a universal human experience, and yet is often a topic clinicians and the general public are not well versed in. Grief brings painful yet entirely natural emotions and physical experiences, which people can heal and grow through. So, the role of the mental or primary care health professional is usually supportive, helping patients to process the loss and to heal. In other words, grief is not generally a pathological experience unless particular vulnerabilities are exacerbated.

The death of a loved one by any cause can be a profoundly painful experience; losing a loved one to suicide comes with layers of additional complexities, which can make suicide bereavement quite unique and extremely painful. While grief is a common human experience, most grief experiences do not require clinical intervention. Many times acute grief naturally transitions to integrated grief – this "healing" being marked by the individual's own recognition of having worked through grief, being able to think of the deceased with equanimity, being able to return to work, to experience pleasure, and to be able to seek companionship and the love of others.[2] However, just as stresses and losses of other kinds can precipitate depression or PTSD in a vulnerable individual, so can the death of a loved one. It is important to keep in mind that depression, anxiety disorders, PTSD, and/or substance misuse can co-occur with grief, and if unaddressed can significantly impede the natural process of healing from loss, leading to much greater disability and negative health outcomes.

C Suicide Bereavement

Losing someone to suicide is a particularly painful and complex type of loss. One way suicide-related grief differs from other types of loss has to do with the way their loved one died and the questions and emotions their loved one's death by suicide evokes. Natural questions of **why** compound a baseline foundational knowledge that may be low concerning suicide in general. In an effort to make sense of the inexplicable and shocking event that has occurred, people generally automatically go into an intense search for information and hypothesis generating. This can lead to guilt, blame, anger at oneself, others, and the loved one who died. This is a natural part of suicide grief, often extremely intense in the initial several months, and often lessening in intensity in the second year and beyond.

● Role of Stigma

Stigma is not to be underestimated as an additional layer that makes suicide bereavement more challenging. While most bereaved families receive an outpouring of support from community, there is often silence when the community members may not have had education to dispel myths concerning suicide, and when the social norms had been exceedingly harsh and discriminating in the historical past. For example, within the current lifetime of people alive today, it was not uncommon for families whose loved one took their life to be shunned in various ways, excommunicated by the church, or the deceased denied a proper burial, and in many places in the world suicide was, or is, a crime, punishable by law.

● Understanding Suicide Helps Loss Survivors

We now have the science to realize suicide is better understood as a succumbing to intense health problems, where someone falls victim to the complex interaction between suffering, health, genetic, social, and environmental factors. And in some (rarer) cases of suicide, it is clear that the mental health condition could be understood similarly to the way one thinks of terminal disease – when even in the face of the best clinical treatment, self-strategies, and family support, like some forms of cancer or other terminal illness, the illness persists, proves to be recalcitrant and malignant, and the person does not survive. While the majority of suicides are not so clear cut, having higher degrees of influence over social and environmental factors in addition to the mental and/or physical health condition(s), we can help people who lose their loved one to suicide by providing this health framework for understanding suicide.

17

● Prevalence and Impact of Suicide Loss

Suicide loss survivors have long been a major force driving the suicide prevention movement forward. And while Dr. Edwin Shneidman described the experience of suicide bereavement and the need for better support resources several decades ago,[3] only in recent years has significant research shed light on the details of prevalence, sequelae, and course of suicide bereavement. A large number of individuals are affected by each suicide death, including family members, friends, colleagues, and others.[4] Therefore a significant portion of community members across multiple countries have been bereaved by suicide at some point during their lifetime. An international meta-analysis of population-based suicide loss studies found 4.3% of community members experienced another's suicide in the past year, and 21.8% during their lifetime.[5] In the USA, even higher rates of exposure were found. From a national sample of 1,432 adults, 51% were suicide exposed and 35% met criteria for suicide bereaved (defined as experiencing moderate to severe emotional distress related to the suicide loss) at some point in their lives.[6] In a sample of 1,736 adults in one state in the USA (Kentucky), 48% had been exposed to suicide loss in their lifetime. Correlating to the degree of perceived closeness to the deceased individual, rates of clinical depression and anxiety disorders were two times greater, and PTSD four times greater, than in suicide unexposed subjects. Suicide exposed individuals were also almost twice as likely to experience suicidal ideation (9% versus 5%)[7] where suicide risk is elevated. There are also increased physical health consequences associated with suicide loss.[8] It is imperative that suicide loss survivors receive the care and support they need to facilitate grieving and prevent any number of significant health risks including increased risk of suicide.

D Terminology

In the past, the commonly used term for survivors of suicide loss had been "Survivors" in suicide prevention circles. However, in recent years as stigma has decreased, an incredibly important point of progress has been people who have survived their own suicide attempt speaking up, advocating for change, and providing a new depth of expertise to the suicide prevention movement. And therefore the more appropriate and clear term for survivors of suicide loss is now "Loss Survivors."

The following are acceptable terms:

- Suicide loss survivors
- Loss survivors
- Survivors of suicide loss
- Persons bereaved by suicide

General Approaches for Patients Bereaved by Suicide

Various interventions have been evaluated for their impact on suicide bereaved people; these include educational and postvention programs at the community level, treatment at the clinical level, and support groups, some of which provide clinical treatment, many of which are considered non-clinical and provide peer support and facilitated processing of grief. All of these interventions, especially those involving the family or community of the bereaved, showed some level of evidence.[9] However, when CG is present, these types of approaches – even treatment of depression – are often not effective.[10,11] All clinicians should receive general education in the experience of suicide bereavement (see AFSP workshop *Suicide Bereavement Clinician Training Program* at afsp.org)[12] and should also be educated about CG.

Clinical Tips for Working with Patients Bereaved by Suicide

An approach to avoid is telling a patient bereaved by suicide that they should be through their grief by now. This is an experience many loss survivors have had with physicians and therapists, and their perception of these words is that the clinician lacks knowledge about the unique features and course of suicide grief, and the overall impact on the treatment relationship can be devastating. Grief is not an experience with an end point, but rather with phases of healing and growth. If you are concerned that there may be comorbid conditions such as depression, PTSD, or CG present, then explain to the patient that for a variety of reasons including prior history, they may be developing an additional condition that actually impedes the process of grief. It is very important to help patients understand you are not going to take their grief away or make them miss their loved one less (they often do not want to let this go), by treating these very serious health conditions. In fact, the patient can expect to continue to grieve and remember their loved one in a way that may feel as intense and intimate, but healthier.

Potential Outcomes Associated with Suicide Bereavement and Recommended Approaches

● Grief in General

When grief is uncomplicated, it is still a painful, often intense, non-linear experience, but is a normal, adaptive response to loss. Noncomplicated grief that is not comorbid with depression does not warrant any formal clinical intervention

17

in most instances. That said, supportive therapy for working through grief – especially after suicide – can be very helpful.[11] Support groups for suicide loss can also be enormously helpful. The International Association of Suicide Prevention (IASP) and AFSP provide many resources for suicide loss survivors; AFSP has a listing of over 500 support groups in the USA. Of course, loss survivors should also receive family and community support as would be the case for any bereaved individuals.

If you have broader connections within the loss survivor's community, encourage community members to shed stigma and approach the person bereaved by suicide just as they would any other person who is grieving. Offering meals, rides, spending time with them, asking if they need help, and if they want to talk about their loved one, should all be encouraged.

● Complicated Grief

In addition to the potential development, recurrence, or worsening of mental health symptoms or conditions, survivors of suicide loss are at increased risk of developing CG. Without specific treatment, CG tends to have a persistent and refractory course. Consider referral to a CGT therapist, or if not available, a therapist who can provide the components of CGT. (See box on CGT components p. 268.) Treat depression or PTSD if present as well.

An estimated 10–20% of bereaved people in the general population (bereaved by any cause of death) experience a more challenging form of grief persisting more than six months beyond the death of their loved one. Among suicide bereaved people the incidence of CG is very high – from 40–80%.[10] CG is characterized by extreme preoccupation and yearning for the deceased person, recurrent painful emotions, ruminations, avoidance of triggers, and difficulty feeling connected to others and their life – a sort of painful acute grief driven "stuckness." It is important to note that CG is essentially synonymous with the newly added Prolonged Grief Disorder in the DSM-5-TR and ICD-11.[13]

Keeping an awareness and vigilance for identifying CG is extremely important since many clinicians mistake it for depression, and depression treatment does not tend to address CG. Distinguishing factors between the two include CG's hallmark features of extreme yearning and overwhelming thoughts about the person the patient lost, whereas depression's hallmark features are sadness and anhedonia that do not necessarily have the extreme longing and obsessional features of

CG. Of course, the two conditions can co-occur, and in that case, both should be addressed, ideally with depression treatment as usual **and** CGT.

Clinical Features of Complicated Grief

Acute grief symptoms that persist for more than six months following the death of a loved one, including:

1. Feelings of intense yearning or longing for the person who died – missing the person so much it is hard to care about anything else

2. Preoccupying memories, thoughts, or images of the deceased person, that may be wanted or unwanted, that interfere with the ability to engage in meaningful activities or relationships with significant others; may include compulsively seeking proximity to the deceased person through pictures, keepsakes, possessions, or other items associated with the loved one

3. Recurrent painful emotions related to the death, such as deep relentless sadness, guilt, envy, bitterness, or anger, that are difficult to control

4. Avoidance of situations, people, or places that trigger painful emotions or preoccupying thoughts related to the death

5. Difficulty restoring the capacity for meaningful positive emotions through a sense of purpose in life, or through satisfaction, joy, or happiness in activities, or relationships with others

CG can be identified reliably using the Inventory of Complicated Grief[14] more than six months after the death of a loved one.

● Treatment for Complicated Grief

Research is clear that CG requires a different approach than uncomplicated grief, but also than depression. While most people with major depression will respond to medication and psychotherapy, CG truly benefits from a more specialized approach, specifically a therapy called Complicated Grief Therapy (CGT).

CGT was developed by Dr. M. Katherine Shear based on attachment theory and interpersonal theory, and has been studied extensively.[16] This treatment combines approaches similar to evidence-based PTSD treatments, interpersonal therapy for grief, and CBT. CGT is generally an individual treatment, although group CGT can also be effective.

17

Key Task Examples in the 16-Week Course of CGT[15,16]

- Facilitate human beings' innate ability to adapt to loss
- Resolve blocks that hinder growth and healing
- Process traumatic aspects of loved one's death
- Strengthen positive emotions and connections with others
- Find a healthy sense of connection to the lost loved one

Strategies in CGT in common with conventional thoughts on dealing with grief include increasing time and activities outside the home, having more interpersonal interactions, and practicing mindfulness-based techniques.

● Depression and PTSD

As discussed above, depression can occur following suicide loss. Resist the common erroneous assumption that any physical or mental health symptoms can be explained by grief and therefore should not be addressed clinically. Be vigilant about depression and PTSD especially in individuals who have a prior history of depression or trauma. Consider medications and/or psychotherapy as indicated for MDD and PTSD. The decision about when to start medication is based on severity, duration, impact, and specific symptoms of depression or PTSD, per usual evaluation and treatment of these conditions. Please see clinical practice guidelines for MDD and PTSD at the American Psychiatric Association and American Psychological Association websites.[17–19] They provide an integrative approach including support, education, cognitive and interpersonal techniques, psychodynamic principles, grief-specific strategies, bright light, exercise, and medication management.

There is no specific or favored medication or therapy for MDD or PTSD in the context of suicide loss, but prior responsiveness to specific medications and their side effect profiles usually provide insight about which medication is best suited for an individual patient.

See the Suicide Loss Support Resource section on p. 277 in the Appendix for resources for patients and families including: a continuously updated list of suicide loss support groups and mental health professionals trained in suicide bereavement, how to request a peer visit from a trained suicide loss survivor, and many more helpful resources.

G — When Healthcare Professionals Lose a Patient to Suicide

This section focuses on the experiences and needs of clinicians who lose a patient to suicide. From the vantage point of the reader, this could encompass their own loss of a patient, it could relate to a clinician patient who has lost a patient, and/or could help the reader in supporting a colleague who has lost a patient.

The loss of a patient or client to suicide can profoundly impact clinicians. There is a fairly robust literature investigating the experiences of mental health professionals' loss of a patient to suicide. Research shows approximately half of psychiatrists and approximately 20% of other mental health professionals experience the loss of one or more patients to suicide over the course of their career.[20] Psychiatry residents are even more likely to experience the suicide of a patient related to the structure of training, with trainees ironically caring for the most severely and chronically ill patient populations.[21] There is scant data about the prevalence of suicide loss experience in primary care and other health disciplines, even though large health system data show health practitioners across most fields take care of patients who die by suicide. Among patients who die by suicide, 60% had been seen by primary care, 40% in an emergency department, and 35% by a mental health professional in the several months prior to their death.[22] It may be the case that these data have not been tracked because suicides and suicidal behavior, until very recent years, have not generally been tracked as clinical outcomes. Thus, when a patient dies by suicide, the primary care provider, cardiologist, or physical therapist for examples, may not even find out about it, whereas, when there is a psychiatrist or psychologist caring for the person, there is a much greater likelihood that the coroner's office or other member of the county's death investigation system would alert the treating clinician or clinic director.

When a clinician loses a patient to suicide, the experience can be far more distressing than one might anticipate, often more similar to the traumatic and profoundly distressing experiences described above for family members than after the loss of patients to physical medical conditions or "natural" causes. For example in one study, half of psychiatrists who lost a patient to suicide had scores on the Impact of an Event Scale comparable to a clinical population after the death of a parent.[23] The loss experience for health professionals also has the challenge of including both personal and professional ramifications.

● Personal Impact

The psychological impact of a patient suicide is variable, but common themes include sadness, shock, anxiety, numbness, anger, and distress; and like personal suicide loss survivors, practitioners often experience an intense retrospective analysis, looking for clues with the benefit of hindsight, and reflecting (or obsessing) on the potential missed opportunities or approaches that could have been different. Fear of culpability, self-blaming, and guilt are common. Posttraumatic experiences including intrusive thoughts, avoidance, and dissociation can also occur. Hendin et al. found half of mental health professionals experienced severe levels of distress for more than one year after the patient death.[24] For many the death of a patient by suicide presents a shift in core beliefs about their own ability to control patient outcomes, and about the very predictability of the world. The opportunity to process these experiences with supervisors and others can facilitate healing and can also lead to posttraumatic growth.[25]

● Professional Issues

Clinicians often have concerns about their clinical care of the deceased patient including their assessment of the patient's suicide risk and missteps in care. Additionally, fears about institutional actions and the potential for a malpractice accusation are common. While suicide is one of the more common reasons for malpractice lawsuits against psychiatrists, they are still quite rare.[26] (See Chapter 11 for details on addressing medicolegal risk after a patient suicide.) Trainees have additional concerns about how the untoward patient outcome could affect their status as a trainee. All levels of experienced clinicians can also have concerns about their colleagues' perceptions. The older prevailing myths about suicide are not exclusive to the non-clinical world; many clinicians had or still have erroneous beliefs about suicide, e.g., that effective clinical care can prevent **all** suicides, rather than decreasing risk, or that with properly formed attachments and rapport in treatment, a patient would not "do that to" their therapist. This self-referential view with exaggerated sense of control is common albeit narcissistic, producing distortion since the patient's risk is actually highly multi-faceted. Strong rapport with a therapist is in fact a protective factor, but other risk factors exist outside clinical care, and acute suffering and cognitive constriction that occurs during the moment of crisis may overwhelm the protective impact of care.

Additionally, conflating suicide prevention with prediction has long plagued the field, and can be seen after patient suicide in contradistinction with the oncologist's reaction to patient loss to cancer or with the cardiologist's after patient death by myocardial infarction. Of course there are overlaps between responses to different causes of patient death, certainly with feelings of grief and concerns about the clinical care that was provided on the minds of other fields' clinicians. But the acknowledgment that outstanding clinical care for cancer and heart disease will not prevent every patient's death is solid for these fields. Science-informed ways of understanding suicide as a complex health outcome have yet to fully take root. Thus when it comes to patient suicide, we are still in a transition phase of science permeating our working model of these complex health outcomes as having multiple underpinnings so that suicide is understood in a similar multifactorial fashion as cancer and heart disease mortality. Even though suicide can be prevented (from a population, public health perspective, or risk-reducing sense for individual patients) that does not mean we can predict suicide. And it does not mean we do not hold ourselves as health professionals to standards of care – we do, with the knowledge that individual patients and illnesses have varying outcomes even with the best clinical care.

Common Experiences after Losing a Patient to Suicide

- Ongoing sense of shame and distress
- Shaken confidence to the point of considering leaving the profession
- Traumatic impact affecting sleep and other aspects of health
- Changes in patient care, hypervigilance with patients, avoidance of certain patients
- Practice management including avoidance of perceived risky patients

Recommended Strategies for Clinicians Who Experience the Suicide of a Patient

- If you are an educator involved in training (in a mental health field or primary care):
  - o Incorporate regular education on the topic of suicide prevention including the experience of losing a patient.[27,28]
  - o Incorporate a postvention response protocol, which aims to support the trainee and entire clinical team, and ensures checking in with affected team members periodically over months that follow the loss.[29]
  - o Educate other staff so that a shared knowledge about the range of reactions will help lesser affected staff to have patience and show support for the team members who are more highly affected.

17

- o Ensure organizational leadership sets a supportive tone for staff and trainees related to critical incidents including patient death by suicide.
- If the clinician is your patient:
  - o Provide empathy and support.
  - o Consider other previous trauma or vulnerabilities which increase likelihood of more severe reactions after patient suicide.
  - o Offer ways for the patient to work through the complicated set of experiences such as time to talk with you, a referral to therapy, or suggesting they discuss their experiences with a trusted mentor.
  - o Continue to check in with your patient about this, in addition to any other active health issues.
  - o Provide your clinician patient with educational resources.[30]
- If you have lost a patient to suicide:
  - o Avail yourself of a supportive process such as debriefing and therapy, as needed over weeks to months.
  - o Practice self-care related to sleep, exercise, substance use, and time for reflection.
  - o Participate in institutional processes such as case review, sentinel event, and root cause analyses.
  - o Meet with risk management.
  - o Offer to meet with the deceased patient's family. This meeting has a clear purpose and parameters – to listen and provide support and empathy for the family, answer questions without violating patient confidentiality, and to offer sincere condolences.
  - o Know that you are not alone in this experience.

KEY TAKEAWAYS

a. Grief is a universal human experience and yet individual experiences are variable and not clinically intuitive. Avoid pathologizing patients' grief experiences; support patients fully, validating their experiences, but also recognizing when symptom severity interferes with healing or life roles.

b. Suicide loss is a profoundly impactful, traumatizing experience for many. It is important that clinicians across specialty areas appreciate the complexities and do not assume that patients' grief has a timeline or a conclusion. Never judge a patient's grief for the timeline or symptoms; rather use therapeutic empathy to support the treatment plan.

c. Help your suicide loss survivor patient by helping them understand more about suicide, for example that suicide risk is multi-faceted and highly complex.

d. Remember that the loved one who died by suicide and their memory can be integrated into one's life moving forward, but people do not "get over" the loss of a loved one.

e. Suicide loss has several known associated potential health outcomes affecting both physical and mental health, as well as increasing suicide risk for some.

f. Provide a balanced assessment of grief-related symptoms: Treat symptoms supportively, such as treating insomnia or agitation for limited periods of time.

g. Monitor for the possible development of depression, PTSD, or Complicated Grief, which occurs in many people bereaved by suicide. Recommended, evidence-based treatment for CG is CGT.

h. Other health sequelae of suicide loss (physical and mental health changes) should be vigilantly screened for and addressed.

i. Clinicians who lose a patient to suicide can have personal and professional impacts that can be mitigated and addressed. If you have lost a patient to suicide, learn more about common reactions, reach out to peers/mentors for support, and consider meeting with a mental health professional for additional debriefing and support.

17

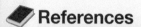

References

1 Neimeyer, R. (Ed.) (2016) *Techniques of Grief Therapy*. New York: Routledge, doi .org/10.4324/9781315692401

2 Zisook, S., & Shear, K. (2009) Grief and bereavement: What psychiatrists need to know. *World Psychiatry: Official Journal of the World Psychiatric Association (WPA)*, 8(2): 67–74. doi: 10.1002/j.2051-5545.2009.tb00217.x

3 Shneidman, E. S. (1973) *Deaths of Man*. New York: Quadrangle.

4 Berman, A. L. (2011) Estimating the population of survivors of suicide: Seeking an evidence base. *Suicide Life Threat Behav*, 41: 110–16. doi: 10.1111/j.1943-278X.2010.00009.x

5 Feigelman, W., Cerel, J., McIntosh, J. L., Brent, D., & Gutin, N. (2017) Suicide exposures and bereavement among American adults: Evidence from the 2016 General Social Survey. *J Affect Disord*, 227: 1–6.

6 Cerel, J., Maple, M., van de Veene, J., Moore, M., Flaherty, C., & Brown, M. (2016) Suicide exposure in the community: Prevalence and correlates in one US state. *Public Health Reports*, 131: 100–7.

7 Crosby, A. E. & Sacks, J. J. (2002) Exposure to suicide: Incidence and association with suicidal ideation and behavior: United States, 1994. *Suicide Life Threat Behav*, 32: 321–8. doi: 10.1521/suli.32.3.321.22170

8 Erlangsen, A., Runeson, B., Bolton, J. M., et al. (2017) Association between spousal suicide and mental, physical, and social health outcomes: a longitudinal and nationwide register-based study. *JAMA Psychiatry*, 74(5): 456–64. psycnet.apa.org/record/2017–19566-002

9 Andriessen, K., Krysinska, K., Hill, N., et al. (2019) Effectiveness of interventions for people bereaved through suicide: a systematic review of controlled studies of grief, psychosocial and suicide-related outcomes. *BMC Psychiatry*, 19(1): 49. doi: 10.1186/s12888-019-2020-z

10 Tal Young, I., Iglewicz, A., Glorioso, D., et al. (2012) Suicide bereavement and complicated grief. *Dialogues in Clinical Neuroscience*, 14(2): 177–86.

11 Zisook, S., & Shuchter, S. (1996) Psychotherapy of the depressions in spousal bereavement. In Session: *Psychotherapy in Practice*. 2: 31–45.

12 American Foundation for Suicide Prevention website. Clinician Training Program on Suicide Bereavement. afsp.org/our-work/loss-healing/suicide-bereavement-clinician-training-program/. Accessed February 29, 2020.

13 American Psychiatric Association. (2013) *Diagnostic and Statistical Manual of Mental Disorders*, 5th ed. Washington, DC: APA Press.

14 Prigerson, H. G., Maciejewski, P. K., Reynolds, C. F., et al. (1995). Inventory of Complicated Grief: A scale to measure maladaptive symptoms of loss. *Psychiatry Res*, 59: 65–79.

15 Shear, M. K. (2015) Clinical practice: Complicated grief. *N Engl J Med*, 372: 153–60.

16 Shear, K., Frank, E., Houck, P. R., & Reynolds, C. F. (2005) Treatment of Complicated Grief: A randomized controlled trial. *JAMA*, 293(21): 2601–8. doi: 10.1001/jama.293.21.2601

17 American Psychiatric Association. (2010) Practice Guideline for the treatment of patients with major depressive disorder. *Am J Psychiatry*, 167(Suppl): 1–118.

18 **American Psychiatric Association Guideline Watch. (2009)** Practice Guideline for the Treatment of Patients with Acute Stress Disorder and Posttraumatic Stress Disorder. Retrieved from psychiatryonline.org/pb/assets/raw/sitewide/practice_guidelines/guidelines/acutestressdisorderptsd-watch.pdf

19 **American Psychological Association. (2017)** Clinical Practice Guideline for the Treatment of Posttraumatic Stress Disorder. Retrieved from www.apa.org/ptsd-guideline/treatments

20 **Ruskin, R., Sakinofsky, I., Bagby, R. M., Dickens, S., & Sousa, G. (2004)** Impact of patient suicide on psychiatrists and psychiatric trainees. *Acad Psychiatry*, 28(2): 104–10.

21 **Leaune, E., Ravella, N., Vieux, M., Poulet, E., Chauliac, N., & Terra, J.-L. (2019)** Encountering patient suicide during psychiatric training: An integrative, systematic review. *Harvard Review of Psychiatry*, 27(3): 141–9. doi: 110.1097/HRP.0000000000000208

22 **Luoma, J. B., Martin, C. E., & Peason, J. L., (2002).** Contact with mental health and primary care providers before suicide: A review of the evidence. *Am J Psychiatry*, 159(6): 909–16.

23 **Chemtob, C. M., Hamada, R. S., Bauer, G., Kinney, B., & Torigoe, R. Y. (1988)** Patients' suicides: Frequency and impact on psychiatrists. *Am J Psychiatry*, 145(2): 224–8.

24 **Hendin, H., Lipschitz, A., Maltsberger, J. T., Haas, A. P., & Wynecoop, S. (2000)** Therapists' reactions to patients' suicides. *Am J Psychiatry*, 157: 2022–7.

25 **Gutin, N. J. (2019)** Losing a patient to suicide: What we know. Part 1. *Current Psychiatry*, 18(10): 14–16, 19–22, 30–32. www.mdedge.com/psychiatry/article/208751/losing-patient-suicide-what-we-know

26 **Jena, A. B., Seabury, S., Lakdawalla, D., & Chandra, A. (2011)** Malpractice risk according to physician specialty. *N Engl J Med*, 365: 629–36.

27 **Prabhakar, D., Anzia, J. M., Balon, R., et al. (2013)** "Collateral damages": Preparing residents for coping with patient suicide. *Acad Psychiatry*, 37(6): 429–30.

28 **Lerner, U., Brooks, K., McNeil, D. E., Cramer, R. J., & Haller, E. (2012)** Coping with a patient's suicide: A curriculum for psychiatry residency training programs. *Acad Psychiatry*, 36(1): 29–33.

29 **Sung, J. C. (2016)** Sample agency practices for responding to client suicide. Forefront: Innovations in Suicide Prevention. Retrieved from www.sprc.org/resources-programs/sample-agency-practices-responding-client-suicide.

30 **McIntosh, J. L. (2019)** Clinicians as survivors of suicide: bibliography. American Association of Suicidology Clinician Survivor Task Force. Retrieved from pages.iu.edu/~jmcintos/Surv.Ther.bib.htm.

Crisis Support Available 24/7 for Yourself or if You Are Worried about Someone Else

o Country-specific resources
   www.iasp.info/resources/Crisis_Centres/

o In the USA to talk by phone: The National Suicide Prevention Lifeline (1–800-273-TALK), veterans press 1
   To chat online https://suicidepreventionlifeline.org/
   Veterans crisis line: www.veteranscrisisline.net/

o In the UK, call, chat, or email Samaritans
   www.samaritans.org/how-we-can-help/contact-samaritan/

o In the USA, Ireland, and Canada to text with a trained counselor: Crisis Text Line (Text TALK to 741741)
   www.crisistextline.org/

o LBGT specialized: The Trevor Project phone or text 1–866-488–7386
   www.thetrevorproject.org/

o Trans Lifelines (USA and Canada): In the USA 1–800-565–8860; In Canada 1–800-330–6366

o Youth country-specific hotlines and resources https://13reasonswhy.info/

For Patients and Family Members: Suicide Prevention Resources

o Suicide warning signs
   https://afsp.org/risk-factors-and-warning-signs
   www.veteranscrisisline.net/SignsOfCrisis/Identifying.aspx
   www.sprc.org/

o Youth specific warning signs
   www.youthsuicidewarningsigns.org/healthcare-professionals

o Steps to take if concerned about someone's mental health or suicide risk
https://afsp.org/find-support/when-someone-is-at-risk/
www.samhsa.gov/find-help

o Information for patients and family members after a suicide attempt
https://afsp.org/find-support/ive-made-attempt/after-an-attempt/
https://afsp.org/find-support/my-loved-one-made-attempt/
www.speakingofsuicide.com/
https://suicidepreventionlifeline.org/help-yourself/attempt-survivors/
https://suicidology.org/resources/suicide-attempt-survivors/
https://didihirsch.org/services/suicide-prevention/therapy-support/

o Treatments specific to reducing suicide risk
https://afsp.org/learn-the-facts

o For members of the public to learn specific techniques that can reduce risk
www.nowmattersnow.org/

o Advocacy opportunities to become a suicide prevention field advocate in the USA
https://afsp.org/our-work/advocacy/become-an-advocate/

o For current suicide statistics in the USA https://afsp.org/suicide-statistics
For suicide rates globally www.who.int/gho/mental_health/suicide_rates/en/

Suicide Loss Support

o For support following the loss of a family member/friend/colleague to suicide
https://afsp.org/find-support/ive-lost-someone/

o Recommended books for suicide loss
https://afsp.org/find-support/ive-lost-someone/resources-loss-survivors/books-loss-survivors/

o To find a suicide loss support group
https://afsp.org/find-support/ive-lost-someone/find-a-support-group/

For Patients and Family Members: Mental Health Resources

o Learn more about mental health conditions
www.nimh.nih.gov/health/topics/index.shtml
www.nami.org/Learn-More/Mental-Health-By-the-Numbers
www.mentalhealthamerica.net/issues/state-mental-health-america

o   For mental health conditions in youth
    www.aacap.org/aacap/families_and_youth/Resource_Centers/Home.aspx
o   Find treatment for a mental health condition
    https://findtreatment.samhsa.gov/locator
    www.mentalhealthamerica.net/finding-help
    https://adaa.org/finding-help/treatment
o   Find treatment for alcohol and other substance use disorders
    https://alcoholtreatment.niaaa.nih.gov/
    Alcohol Use Disorder Treatment Services UK
    www.nhs.uk/live-well/alcohol-support/
    Drug Addiction Services UK
    www.nhs.uk/live-well/healthy-body/drug-addiction-getting-help/
o   Peer support
    www.dbsalliance.org/site/PageServer?pagename=peer_landing
o   About mental health treatments
    www.nimh.nih.gov/health/publications/index.shtml
    www.mentalhealthamerica.net/issues/state-mental-health-america
o   About treatment for children
    www.aacap.org/aacap/families_and_youth/resource_centers/Home.aspx
    www.nimh.nih.gov/health/publications/treatment-of-children-with-mental-illness-fact-sheet/index.shtml
o   For parents or adults working with LGBTQ youth familyproject.sfsu.edu
o   For parents on children and teens' mental health and suicide prevention
    https://afsp.org/campaigns/talk-about-mental-health-awareness/teens-and-suicide-what-parents-should-know/
o   Help a peer in high school or college
    www.jedfoundation.org/mental-health-resource-center/
    https://seizetheawkward.org/
o   Mental health advocacy
    https://mhaadvocate.com/
    www.nami.org/Get-Involved/Take-Action-on-Advocacy-Issues

o To consider participating in a clinical trial
www.nimh.nih.gov/health/trials/index.shtml

Occupation-Specific Suicide Prevention Resources

o Workplace Suicide Prevention
https://theactionalliance.org/communities/workplace

o USA Department of Defense Military
www.dspo.mil/

o Construction
www.cfma.org/news/content.cfm?ItemNumber=4570

o Law Enforcement
www.policeforum.org/assets/PreventOfficerSuicide.pdf

https://bluehelp.org/

o Farm and Agricultural Workers
www.farmaid.org/

o Physician and Healthcare Professionals
AFSP https://afsp.org/our-work/education/healthcare-professional-burnout-depression-suicide-prevention/

ACGME www.acgme.org/What-We-Do/Initiatives/Physician-Well-Being/Resources

AMA Suicide Prevention for Physicians www.stepsforward.org/modules/preventing-physician-suicide

www.dentistrytoday.com/news/todays-dental-news/item/1098-suicide-and-dentistry-myths-realities-and-prevention

Nursing Suicide Prevention https://www.nursingworld.org/practice-policy/nurse-suicide-prevention/

Veterinary Medicine Professionals
www.avma.org/ProfessionalDevelopment/PeerAndWellness/Pages/get-help.aspx

Clinical Resources: Suicide Screening, Assessment, Clinical Guidelines

o Recommended clinical standards for preventing patient suicide
https://theactionalliance.org/resource/recommended-standard-care
www.jointcommission.org/resources/patient-safety-topics/suicide-prevention

o The Joint Commission Suicide Prevention Portal
www.jointcommission.org/topics/suicide_prevention_portal.aspx

o Screening Pathway (Adult and Youth Clinical Pathways for Inpatient, Outpatient, Emergency Department)
   www.nimh.nih.gov/ASQ

o Columbia Lighthouse Project
   "cssrs.columbia.edu/"

o Guidelines/pocket guide for suicide risk assessment
   o SAMHSA https://store.samhsa.gov/product/SAFE-T-Pocket-Card-Suicide-Assessment-Five-Step-Evaluation-and-Triage-for-Clinicians/sma09-4432
   o Veterans Administration www.mentalhealth.va.gov/docs/va029assessmentguide.pdf

o Clinical practice guidelines related to major psychiatric conditions
   o American Psychiatric Association Clinical Practice Guidelines
   www.psychiatry.org/psychiatrists/practice/clinical-practice-guidelines

o Professional organizations that provide suicide prevention education
   o American Foundation for Suicide Prevention (AFSP)
      https://afsp.org/take-action/get-training/
   o SafeSide Suicide Prevention Training for Clinicians
      www.safesideprevention.com/
   o Collaborative Assessment and Management of Suicidality
      https://cams-care.com/
   o Suicide Prevention Resource Center
      www.sprc.org/training
   o The American Psychiatric Association (APA)
      http://psychiatryonline.org/pb/assets/raw/sitewide/practice_guidelines/guidelines/suicide-guide.pdf
   o The American Psychological Association
      www.apa.org/topics/suicide/
   o American Association of Suicidology (AAS)
      www.suicidology.org/training-accreditation/rrsr
   o American Academy of Pediatrics (AAP)
      aap.org
   o International Association for Suicide Prevention (IASP)
      www.iasp.info/

- o International Academy of Suicide Research (IASR)
  https://suicide-research.org
- o Association for Death Education and Counseling (ADEC)
  www.adec.org/
- o The Samaritans
  https://samaritanshope.org/get-help/
- o Jed Foundation
  www.jedfoundation.org/
- o Healthcare System Framework
  - o Zero Suicide
    http://zerosuicide.edc.org/
  - o SafeSide
    www.safesideprevention.com/
  - o Collaborative Assessment and Management of Suicidality
    https://cams-care.com/
- o Treating Suicidal Patients via Telemedicine/Telehealth Services
  https://theactionalliance.org/sites/default/files/covid-suicidescreentelehealth.pdf and
  www.nimh.nih.gov/research/research-conducted-at-nimh/asq-toolkit-materials/
  inpatient/covid-19-adult-clinical-pathway-chart-description.shtml
  www.sprc.org/resources-programs/treating-suicidal-patients-during-covid-19

Clinical Resources: Support for Clinicians After Patient Suicide

- o SPRC
  www.sprc.org/resources-programs/clinicians-survivors-after-suicide-loss
- o AFSP Clinician Suicide Bereavement Training
  https://afsp.org/suicide-bereavement-clinician-training

Clinical Pediatric Resources

- o UCLA–Duke Center for Suicide, Self-harm and Substance Abuse Treatment and
  Prevention: Act Support and Protect (ASAP Center)
  www.asapnctsn.org/what-we-do/

  To learn more about suicide prevention evidence-based treatment modalities

o AACAP Resources for Primary Care
www.aacap.org/AACAP/Resources_for_Primary_Care/Home.aspx

o AAP Suicide Prevention Resources
www.aap.org/en-us/about-the-aap/aap-press-room/campaigns/suicide-prevention/Pages/default.aspx

Community, School, and Workplace Suicide Prevention Resources

- Prevention
  - o K-12 Model school district policy for suicide prevention
    https://afsp.org/our-work/education/model-school-policy-suicide-prevention/
  - o For colleges and universities
    jedfoundation.org
  - o Comprehensive blueprint for workplace suicide prevention
    www.sprc.org/settings/workplaces
- Postvention: actions to take following a suicide
  - o After a suicide: a toolkit for schools (K-12)
    https://afsp.org/our-work/education/after-a-suicide-a-toolkit-for-schools/
  - o Postvention: a guide for response to suicide on college campuses
    https://hemha.org/wp-content/uploads/2018/06/jed-hemha-postvention-guide.pdf
  - o After a medical resident/fellow suicide: a toolkit for residency programs
    https://chapterland.org/wp-content/flipbooks/physiciantoolkit/inc/pdf/flipbook.pdf
  - o After a suicide: a toolkit for medical schools
    https://chapterland.org/wp-content/uploads/sites/13/2018/09/13719_AFSP_Medical_School_Toolkit_m1_v3.pdf
  - o After a suicide in the workplace
    https://theactionalliance.org/communities/workplace

Index

Locators in **bold** refer to tables; those in *italic* to figures